Official Organ of the European Society for [illegible] Endocrinology

Hormone Research

International Journal of Experimental and Clinical Endocrinology

Founded 1970 as 'Hormones' by M. Marois

KARGER

Printed in Switzerland
on acid-free paper by
Thür AG Offsetdruck, Pratteln

Appears monthly:
2 volumes per year (12 issues)

Hormone Research

'Hormone Research' aims to provide rapid publication of clinical investigations and case reports, as well as experimental and methodological work related to endocrinology. Correspondence is welcome, but publication of letters is at the discretion of the editors.

Submission: Only original papers written in English are considered and should be sent to:

S. Karger AG
Editorial Dept. 'Hormone Research'
P.O. Box
CH-4009 Basel (Switzerland)

Manuscripts should be submitted in triplicate (with three sets of illustrations of which one is an original), typewritten double-spaced on one side of the paper, with a wide margin.

Conditions: All manuscripts are subject to editorial review. Manuscripts are received with the explicit understanding that they are not under simultaneous consideration by any other publication. Submission of an article for publication implies the transfer of the copyright from the author to the publisher upon acceptance. Accepted papers become the permanent property of 'Hormone Research' and may not be reproduced by any means, in whole or in part, without the written consent of the publisher. It is the author's responsibility to obtain permission to reproduce illustrations, tables, etc. from other publications.

Arrangement:
Title page: The first page of each paper should indicate the title (main title underlined), the authors' names, and the institute where the work was conducted. A short title for use as running head as well as the full address of the author to whom correspondence should be sent are also required.
Full address: The exact postal address complete with postal code must be given at the bottom of the title page. Please also supply Phone and Fax numbers.
Key words: For indexing purposes, a list of 3-10 key words in English is essential.
Abstract: Each paper needs an abstract of up to 10 lines.
Small type: Paragraphs which can or must be set in smaller type (case histories, test methods, etc.) should be indicated with a 'p' (petit) in the margin on the left-hand side.
Footnotes: Avoid footnotes. When essential, they are numbered consecutively and typed at the foot of the appropriate page.
Tables and illustrations: Tables and illustrations (both numbered in Arabic numerals) should be prepared on separate sheets. Tables require a heading and figures a legend, also prepared on a separate sheet. For the reproduction of illustrations, only good drawings and original photographs can be accepted; negatives or photocopies cannot be used. When possible, group several illustrations on one block for reproduction (max. size 181 × 223 mm) or provide crop marks. On the back of each illustration, indicate its number, the author's name, and 'top'. Color illustrations are reproduced at the author's expense.
References: In the text identify references by Arabic numerals [in square brackets]. Material submitted for publication but not yet accepted should be noted as 'unpublished data' and not be included in the reference list. The list of references should include only those publications which are cited in the text. Do not alphabetize; number references in the order in which they are first mentioned in the text. The surnames of the authors followed by initials should be given. There should be no punctuation other than a comma to separate the authors. Cite all authors, 'et al' is not sufficient. Abbreviate journal names according to the Index Medicus system. (Also see International Committee of Medical Journal Editors: Uniform requirements for manuscripts submitted to biomedical journals. Br Med J 1988;296:401-405.)
Examples
(a) Papers published in periodicals: Kauffman HF, van der Heide S, Beaumont F, Blok H, de Vries K: Class-specific antibody determination against *Aspergillus fumigatus* by means of the enzyme-linked immunosorbent assay. III. Comparative study: IgG, IgA, IgM ELISA titers, precipitating antibodies and IgE binding after fractionation of the antigen. Int Arch Allergy Appl Immunol 1986;80:300-306.
(b) Monographs: Matthews DE, Farewell VT: Using and Understanding Medical Statistics. Basel, Karger, 1985.
(c) Edited books: Hardy WD Jr, Essex M: FeLV-induced feline acquired immune deficiency syndrome: A model for human AIDS;in Klein E (ed): Acquired Immunodeficiency Syndrome. Prog Allergy. Basel, Karger, 1986, vol 37, pp 353-376.
Further details: Authors may consult our leaflet 'Rules for the Preparation of Manuscripts', available on request from the Publisher, S. Karger AG, P.O. Box, CH-4009 Basel (Switzerland).

Page charges: There is no page charge for papers of 4 or fewer printed pages (including tables, illustrations and references). Each additional complete or partial page is charged to the author at SFr. 415.–/ US$ 275.00. The allotted size of a paper is equal to approx. 12 manuscript pages (including tables, illustrations and references). As the page charges are waived in any case for the first paper each year to be published by a member of ESPE, authors who are members of the ESPE should so indicate on the title page.

Galley proofs: Unless indicated otherwise, galley proofs are sent to the first-named author and should be returned with the least possible delay. Alterations made in galley proofs, other than the correction of printer's errors, are charged to the author. No page proofs are supplied.

Reprints: Order forms and a price list are sent with the galley proofs. Orders submitted after the issue is printed are subject to considerably higher prices. Allow five weeks from date of publication for delivery of reprints.

KARGER

General Information

Hormone Research

Publication data: 'Hormone Research' is published 12 times annually. Volumes 37–38 with 6 issues each appear in 1992

Subscription rates: Subscriptions run for a full calendar year. Prices are given per volume, surface postage included.

Personal subscription: SFr. 278.60, US$ 186.20. (Must be in the name of, billed to, and paid by an individual. Order must be marked 'personal subscription'.)

Institutional subscription:
(Regular rate.) SFr. 398.–, US$ 266.00.

Members of the European Society of Paediatric Endocrinology: SFr. 76.40, US$ 51.05.
Lawson Wilkins Society; ISGD; Schweizerische Gesellschaft für Endokrinologie: SFr. 238.80, US$ 159.60.

Airmail postage: SFr. 35.–, US$ 30.00. (Extra per volume.)

Microform subscription: SFr. 199.–, US$ 133.00. (Available exclusively to subscribers of the paper edition.)

Single issues and back volumes: Information on availability and prices can be obtained through the Publisher.

Advertising: Correspondence and rate requests should be addressed to the Publisher.

Subscription orders: Orders can be placed at agencies, bookstores, directly with the Publisher S. Karger AG, P.O. Box, CH – 4009 Basel (Switzerland) or with any of the following distributors:

Deutschland:
S. Karger GmbH, Lörracher Strasse 16A
Postfach, D-W–7800 Freiburg

France: Librairie Luginbühl
36, bd de Latour-Maubourg, F–75007 Paris

Great Britain, Ireland:
S. Karger Publishers, 11 Ravenscroft Road
Beckenham, Kent BR3 4TP

USA: S. Karger Publishers, Inc.
26 West Avon Road, P.O. Box 529
Farmington, CT 06085

India, Bangladesh, Sri Lanka:
S. Karger India Subscription Agency
B – 5/132 Safdarjung Enclave
New Delhi-110029

Japan: Katakura Libri, Inc.
36-9 Hongo 3-chome, Bunkyo-ku, Tokyo 113

Change of address: Both old and new address should be stated and sent to the subscription source.

Bibliographic indices: This journal is regularly listed in bibliographic services, including *Current Contents®*.

Book Reviews: Books are accepted for review by special agreement.

Guidelines for Disk Submission

Karger Publishers welcomes the submission of manuscripts on disk.

Please observe the 'Instructions to authors' as well as the following guidelines:

Technical Data

The preferred **storage medium** is a 3.5- or 5.25-inch disk in MS-DOS format. Macintosh is also acceptable.

The preferred **word processing package** is Microsoft Word. Other commonly used PC text programs are also accepted, as well as ASCII formats.

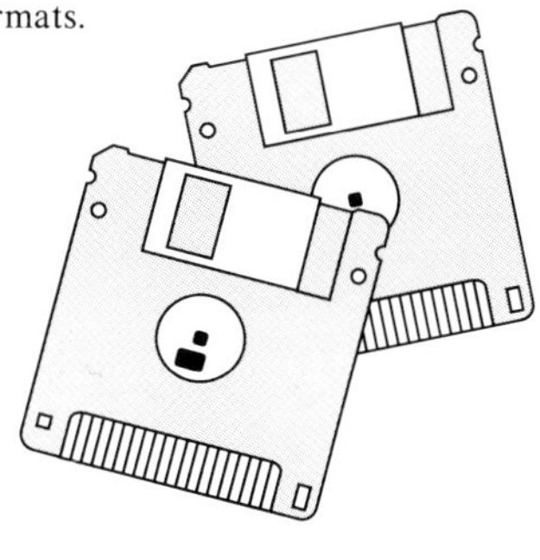

Handling

All manuscripts accepted for Karger publications are subject to copy editing. It is therefore essential that you send us a **double-spaced printout** of your manuscript which exactly matches the disk.

Any subsequent revised versions should be clearly marked as such, both on the disk and on the manuscript.

The copy-edited manuscript and the disk will be returned to you along with the galley proofs. Please be sure to **check the galleys against the manuscript** in which changes introduced by the copy editor and/or questions will be marked.

Please **label** your disk with (a) the title of the journal for which it is submitted, (b) a short version of the paper title, (c) your name and (d) the software and hardware used.

Text Arrangement

Text and headings should be ranged left throughout, without word breaks. **Do not center, space, or use block letters** for text and headings (except for abbreviations).

Do not use indentations to mark the beginning of a paragraph, but use one blank line between paragraphs.

Be sure to use the **same type style for headings of the same ranking** throughout the text.

When using **special characters** not available on a standard keyboard (including Greek characters), please do so by a readily identifiable code, and use the same code throughout the manuscript. Supply a **complete list of the codes used** at the beginning of the text.

Illustrations, tables and mathematical formulae will be handled conventionally.

KARGER

Pediatric and Adolescent Medicine (ISSN 1017–5989), **Vol. 2**
Series Editor: D. Branski, Jerusalem

Editors: P.L. Giorgi, R.M. Suskind, C. Catassi

The Obese Child

A multidisciplinary approach encompassing such areas as genetics, morphology, biochemistry, radiology, psychology and nutrition

Although the life-threatening consequences of obesity are mainly seen during adulthood, it is now clear that obesity-related degenerative diseases, including type II diabetes mellitus, hypertension and atherosclerosis, begin in the first years of life. This book presents an up-to-date review of biological, medical and psychological aspects of childhood obesity from a holistic point of view. Special emphasis is given to problems specific to pediatric obesity such as the development of adipose tissue, metabolic peculiarities, clinical features of syndromic obesity, psychosocial factors and strategies for prevention and treatment. Highlighting recent progress and delineating future research objectives, this volume is important reading for pediatricians, nutritionists, biochemists and psychologists interested in this complex disorder.

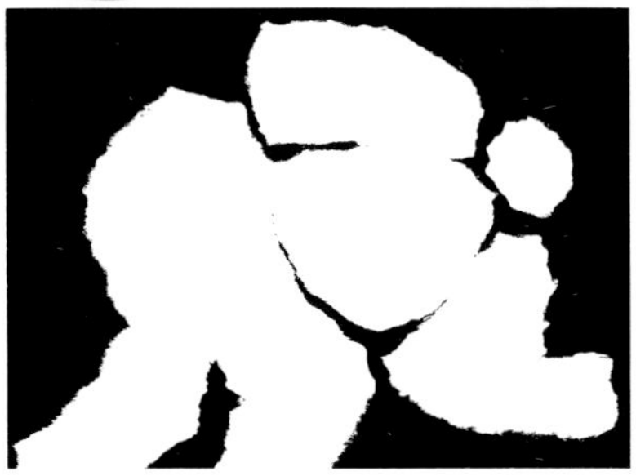

Contents

Fields of Interest
Pediatrics; Nutrition; Biochemistry, Endocrinology, Metabolism;
Clinical Nutrition, Dietetics, Genetics, Preventive Medicine, Psychology

Pediatric and Adolescent Medicine, Vol. 2
The Obese Child
Meeting of the Department of Pediatrics, University of Ancona, Ancona, September 1990
Editors: Giorgi, P.L. (Ancona); Suskind, R.M. (New Orleans, La.); Catassi, C. (Ancona)
VIII + 256 p., 65 fig., 49 tab., hard cover, 1992
SFr. 231.– / DM 277.– / US $ 185.00
Prices subject to change
DM price for FRG, US $ price for USA only
ISBN 3-8055-5463-X

KI 92522

KARGER

Hormonal Resistance Syndromes

35th International
Henri-Pierre Klotz Symposium on
Hormonal Resistance Syndromes,
Paris, May 14–15, 1992

Guest Editors
P. Jaquet and *P. Vague,* Marseille

28 figures, 13 tables, 1992

KARGER

S. Karger
Medical and Scientific Publishers
Basel · Freiburg · Paris · London
New York · New Delhi · Bangkok
Singapore · Tokyo · Sydney

Drug Dosage
The authors and the publisher have exerted every effort to ensure that drug selection and dosage set forth in this text are in accord with current recommendations and practice at the time of publication. However, in view of ongoing research, changes in government regulations, and the constant flow of information relating to drug therapy and drug reactions, the reader is urged to check the package insert for each drug for any change in indications and dosage and for added warnings and precautions. This is particularly important when the recommended agent is a new and/or infrequently employed drug.

Printed in Switzerland on acid-free paper by
Thür AG Offsetdruck, Pratteln
ISBN 3–8055–5784–1

Contents

Horm Res 1992;38:5–12

E. Clauser
I. Leconte
C. Auzan

INSERM U36, Collège de France, Paris, France

Molecular Basis of Insulin Resistance

Key Words
Insulin resistance
Insulin
Insulin receptor
Mutation
Gene polymorphism
Cellular signalling
Phosphorylation
Glucose transporter

Abstract
The recent application of recombinant DNA technology to clinical investigation now allows the identification of the molecular alterations responsible for insulin resistance. In this review, the recent knowledge concerning these investigations is reported. Genetic mutations of the insulin gene as the source of insulin resistance have been reported for a long time. More recently a series of mutations of the insulin receptor gene have been identified as the cause of the extreme insulin resistance, observed in rare syndromes, such as type A insulin resistance or leprechaunism. However, it is probable that the majority of the molecular defects causing insulin resistance occur at the postreceptor level. The key proteins involved in the different intracellular signalling pathways of insulin are only partly identified. A better understanding of the mechanisms of insulin action is essential for the identification of corresponding genetic alterations. The investigations concerning the glucose transporter GLUT4 and glucokinase genes are good examples of complex but promising research, which has recently started. Elucidation of the genetic and molecular basis of diseases such as type II diabetes or other states associated with insulin resistance, is the long-term goal.

The physiological consequences of an abnormal action of insulin on its target tissues, such as liver, muscles or adipose tissue, are observed in many clinical diseases. This insulin resistance is due to structural or functional defects of different proteins involved in the mechanisms of insulin action and primarily insulin and insulin receptor. The limitation of our understanding of these molecular defects comes essentially from the extreme complexity of the different signalling pathways linking the insulin receptor to the different metabolic effects of insulin within the cell. Although the past few years have seen great progress in the knowledge of these proteins mediating the actions of insulin inside the cell, a complete overview is still impossible.

In parallel to the investigation of the mechanisms of insulin action, the physiological analysis of the causes of insulin resistance states was developed, trying to distinguish between primary (genetic?) and secondary (acquired?) defects and to localize the level(s) (prereceptor, receptor or postreceptor) of the alteration(s).

For those proteins already identified as key proteins of the insulin action, the molecular mutations responsible

E. Clauser
INSERM U36
Collège de France
3, rue d'Ulm
F–75005 Paris (France)

for primary insulin resistance can now be identified with the recently developed tools of molecular biology applied to clinical investigation.

The Molecular Mechanisms of Insulin Action

Insulin

Insulin, secreted by the B cells of the pancreas, is the first key protein of the system. The structures of this protein, its gene and mRNA were elucidated more than 10 years ago [1]. The insulin gene is a 1.5-kbp sequence located in chromosome 11 and includes 3 exons. Exons 2 and 3 code for the preproinsulin containing successively the signal peptide (24 amino acids), the insulin B chain (30 amino acids), the connecting peptide (30 amino acids) and the insulin A chain (20 amino acids). Intracellular cleavage of the signal peptide and the C peptide produces the insulin molecule composed of two chains linked by disulfide bridges. Qualitative alterations of insulin are responsible for insulin resistance.

Insulin Receptor

Insulin acts on its different target tissues through a membrane-bound receptor. This receptor is a glycoprotein coded by a unique gene and belongs to the tyrosine kinase family of receptors [2, 3]. The insulin receptor gene is very long (> 150 kbp), located on chromosome 19 and contains 22 exons [4]. This gene codes for two slightly different proteins composed of an external α subunit of 723 or 735 amino acids and a transmembrane β subunit of 620 amino acids, containing extracellular and transmembrane domains and an intracellular domain, which includes a tyrosine kinase domain. Two different insulin receptor subtypes have been identified, which differ by the presence (type B) or the absence (type A) of a 12 amino acid sequence at the C-terminus of the α subunit, due to an alternate splicing of exon 11. These two subtypes vary in their affinity for insulin [5]. The binding of insulin to the extracellular α subunit results in an activation of the tyrosine kinase of its β subunit, which is the first step of the intracellular modifications leading to the actions of insulin. This key role of the receptor and its tyrosine kinase for insulin actions designated it as a potential target of modifications responsible for insulin resistance.

Intracellular Signalling Pathways

Following insulin receptor tyrosine activation a number of events occur in the cell, which are still not completely understood. The most logical consequence of tyrosine kinase activation is the phosphorylation of cytosolic or membrane-bound substrates. In fact, a lot of different cellular proteins are phosphorylated inside the cell in response to insulin or by the insulin-activated receptor, but the exact role of these proteins, mostly kinases or phosphatases, in insulin actions and the precise order and number of these cascades of phosphorylations are still the subject of many investigations [6]. Serine kinases, which are activated by phosphorylation on tyrosyl residue, are potential candidates. Proteins, the phosphorylation of which is strongly and quickly stimulated after insulin binding, such as pp185 in hepatocytes and pp120, a membrane-bound ATPase or pp15 in adipocytes, were particularly studied [7]. Other key proteins in cellular metabolism have been investigated, such as calmodulin, which is tyrosine phosphorylated in response to insulin. Finally the possibility that some insulin actions are mediated through a pathway involving second messengers such as glycolipids or diacylglycerol has been suggested by some recent experiments [8]. Activation of γ phospholipase C by phosphorylation is the probable link between this signalling pathway and the insulin receptor. In conclusion, some pieces of a complex puzzle have been assembled, but the complete picture of the intracellular signalling pathways of insulin is not yet evident.

The metabolic consequences of insulin binding to the cell surface are multiple and depend on the nature of the target tissue. Many different key enzymes are stimulated or inhibited by insulin (fig. 1). Glucose metabolism is modified by a combined stimulatory effect on glucose transport and glycolysis in all tissues and also glycogen synthesis in the liver, in the muscle and adipose tissue and an inhibitory effect on gluconeogenesis and glycogenolysis in the liver. These physiological effects are the consequences of the activation of the insulin-dependent glucose transporter (GLUT4) and also of multiple enzymes such as glucokinase, glycogen synthase (glycogen synthesis), phosphofructokinase, pyruvate kinase and pyruvate dehydrogenase (glycolysis). Inhibition of hexokinase, glycogen phosphorylase and phosphoenolpyruvate carboxykinase are also observed. In adipose tissue, the lipid synthesis is stimulated by insulin via an activation of citrate lyase, acetyl-CoA carboxylase, fatty acid synthase, glycerol-3-phosphate dehydrogenase and lipoprotein lipase [9]. All these protein activations or inhibitions result from different mechanisms. Activation of the glucose transport results essentially from a translocation of glucose transporters from an intracellular pool to the membrane [10]. Some of these enzymes are activated by phosphorylation

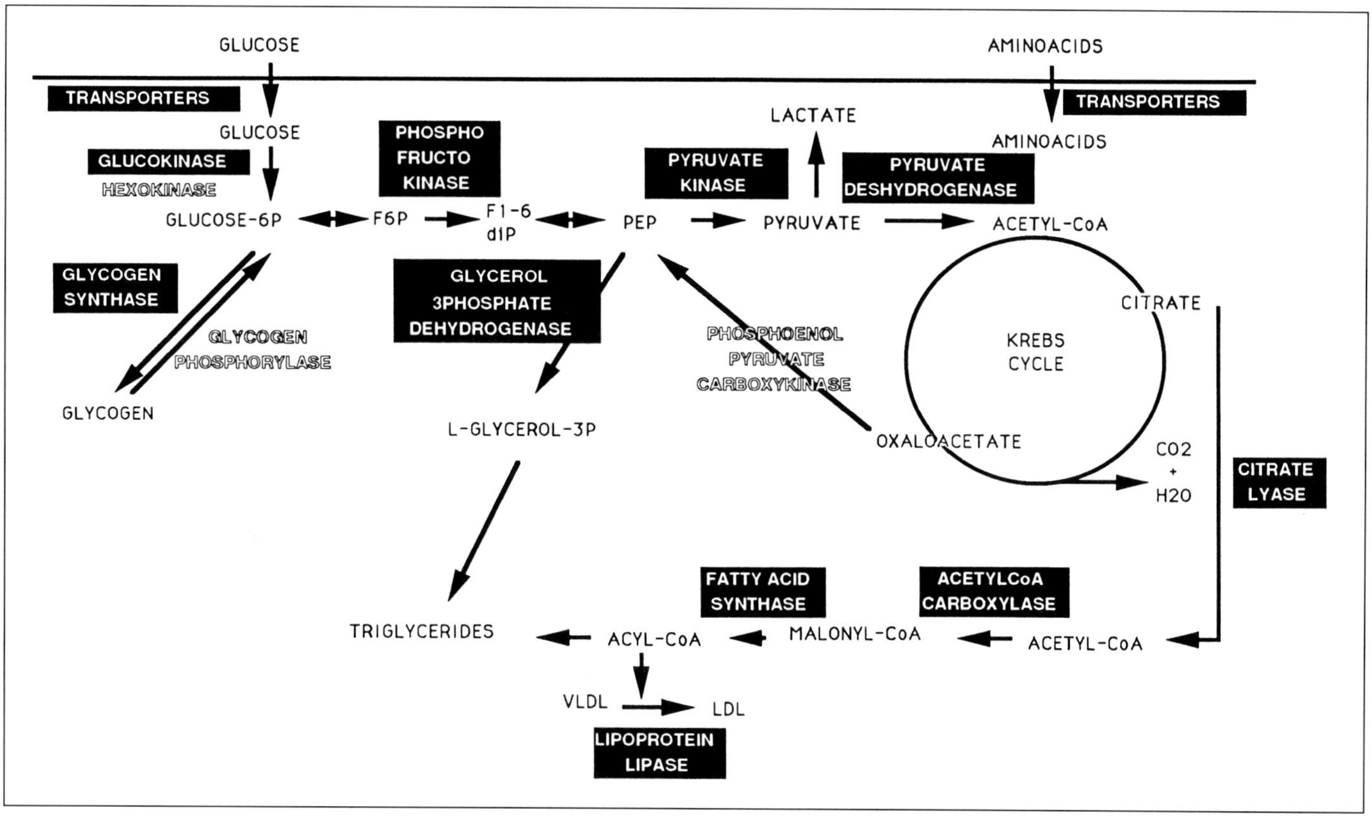

Fig. 1. Schematic representation of glucose and lipid metabolisms inside a hypothetical cell, possessing all the insulin-regulated proteins. Enzymes or transporters, which are stimulated by insulin, are indicated on a black background. Enzymes which are inhibited by insulin are represented in outline style. F6P = Fructose-6-phosphate; F1–6 diP = fructose-1,6-diphosphate; PEP = phosphoenolpyruvate. The upper horizontal line represents the cell membrane.

(acetyl-CoA carboxylase) or dephosphorylation (pyruvate deshydrogenase), but the precise cascade of phospho/dephosphorylation linking the activation of insulin receptor to these enzymes is not known. In other cases the transcription of the genes for these enzymes is modified by insulin. Glucokinase or pyruvate kinase gene transcriptions are stimulated by insulin, whereas phosphoenolpyruvate carboxykinase gene transcription is inhibited. In these cases, phosphorylation of trans-acting factors regulating the gene transcription is the more likely explanation.

This short and not exhaustive description of the different proteins involved in the multiple cellular actions of insulin shows clearly the complexity of the situation. Potentially, every genetic or secondary molecular alteration of each of these key proteins is capable of producing an insulin resistance state. Therefore, the analysis of the molecular defects responsible for insulin resistance is only just beginning.

From Physiological to Clinical Aspects of Insulin Resistance

Physiological Classification of Insulin Resistance

The knowledge of the mechanisms of insulin actions allows the division of the mechanisms of insulin resistance into three groups: prereceptor, receptor and postreceptor insulin resistance [11]. The prereceptor insulin resistance essentially concerns the alterations of insulin structure or function. Qualitative modifications of insulin can follow a genetic mutation of its gene. Anti-insulin antibodies can block the insulin action. Accelerated degradation of insulin can also be responsible for prereceptor insulin resistance.

Receptor insulin resistance is the consequence of a decrease in the number of insulin receptors at the surface of the cells, a reduction in the affinity of the receptor for insulin or a defect in the activation of the tyrosine kinase. These changes in the functions of insulin receptor can be genetically determined or acquired in some pathological situations.

Finally, the majority of insulin resistance is of the postreceptor type, given the extraordinary complexity of the intracellular pathways of insulin action. This insulin resistance is generally identified by default and its molecular basis is poorly understood.

Multiple Clinical Syndromes

Insulin Defects. Structural or functional modifications of insulin are responsible for some cases of insulin resistance. The production of antibodies against insulin is the most classical cause. Mutants of insulin gene have also been described, resulting in either familial hyperproinsulinemia or insulinopathies. In both cases, the level of circulating immunological insulin-like material is extremely high and glycoregulation disorders can be present. A normal sensitivity to exogenous insulin is observed generally. Different mutations of the insulin gene are responsible for either an absence of connecting peptide cleavage, resulting in the production of proinsulin (Ser10 for His and Arg65 for His) or an abnormal insulin (Phe24 for Ser, Phe25 for Leu in the B chain and Val68 for Leu in the A chain) [12].

Insulin Receptor Defects. In parallel to insulin defects, different clinical syndromes may be due to structural or functional modifications of the insulin receptor [13, 14]. The presence of high levels of antibodies against the insulin receptor in the plasma realizes the rare but classical syndrome of type B insulin resistance. This maturity onset insulin resistance occurs essentially in women and is associated with acanthosis nigricans, immunological disorders with extremely high levels of plasma insulin. The diagnosis is obtained by the identification of the antibodies against the insulin receptor.

Structural alterations of the insulin receptor are suspected in different familial diseases with extreme insulin resistance. The role of the insulin receptor was demonstrated by the significant reduction of the number or affinity of these receptors for insulin in some patients. Tyrosine kinase defects were also observed. These extremely rare diseases are of different types:

(a) Type A insulin resistance is the most classical. It occurs in young women, who present with acanthosis nigricans, hyperandrogenism and carbohydrate intolerance. The familial inheritance of insulin resistance and insulin receptor functional abnormalities lead to the conclusion of a possible genetic defect.

(b) Leprechaunism is a malformative syndrome affecting infants with growth retardation, characteristic facial features, hirsutism and major insulin resistance. Insulin-binding properties of the receptors are altered in some but not all leprechaun patients.

(c) Lipoatrophic diabetes is another rare syndrome of extreme insulin resistance. The major clinical features are diabetes, atrophy of the subcutaneous adipose tissue, biologically associated with hypertriglyceridemia. The mechanisms of this syndrome seem to be heterogeneous, since congenital or acquired, complete or partial forms have been described, together with normal or altered functioning of the insulin receptor.

(d) Finally, Rabson-Mendenhall syndrome is another rare congenital disease, which is associated to extreme insulin resistance, adrenal and pineal hyperplasia and abnormalities of the nails and teeth.

All these syndromes have in common a major insulin resistance, abnormal insulin receptor functions in some cases and a genetic determinism, which make them good candidates to be determined by mutations of the insulin receptor gene.

Other Insulin Resistances. Hypersecretions of cortisol, growth hormone, catecholamines and glucagon are all able to produce insulin resistance [14]. Primary (Cushing syndrome, acromegaly, pheochromocytoma or glucagonoma) or secondary (stress, etc.) hyperproductions of these hormones modify the action of insulin. The molecular basis of these antagonistic actions are only partly known and include inhibition of insulin secretion, modifications of insulin receptor, glucose transporter and glucose metabolism key enzymes and substrates.

The most frequent diseases associated with insulin resistance are type II diabetes and obesity [11]. Both population and familial studies indicate that these diseases present hereditary determinants. Therefore, the genetic molecular defects, which initiate the diseases, have been actively investigated. A primary insulin resistance is one hypothesis. Abnormalities of insulin action were demonstrated at the receptor and postreceptor levels. The receptor defects are essentially represented by a decrease in the number of insulin receptors at the surface of the cells, directly linked to the hyperinsulinemia and due to a general physiological mechanism called 'down-regulation'. In type II diabetes a defect of tyrosine kinase activation is also clearly demonstrated. Different postreceptor defects are also suspected in type II diabetes, but their precise molecular nature is unknown. In addition to the insulin resistance, type II diabetic patients usually present a defect in insulin secretion. It is still difficult to identify which of these two abnormalities is primary. There is good evidence that the insulin resistance, observed in

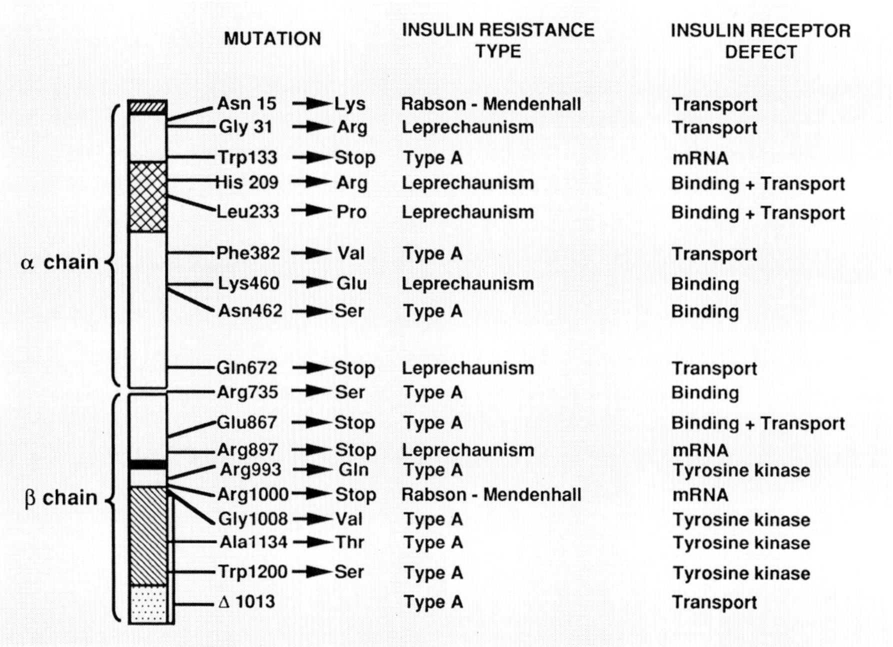

Fig. 2. Representation of the known mutations of the insulin receptor responsible for insulin resistance. On the left is a schematically represented insulin receptor structure, with the α chain containing the signal peptide (▨) and the cross-linking domain (⊠) and the β chain. The β chain includes the transmembrane domain (■), the tyrosine kinase (▧) and the C-terminal domain (▦). The first column (Mutation) shows and localizes the different mutations already identified in families presenting extreme insulin resistance. The wild type amino acid, its position in the sequence [according to 2] and the mutated amino acid are successively indicated. The second column indicates the nature of the clinical insulin resistance syndrome corresponding to the mutation. The last column indicates the nature of the functional alteration of the insulin receptor.

vivo, is reversible in vitro in primary culture, indicating a secondary mechanism. However, in the absence of a clear answer on the nature of the primary defect responsible for the disease and given the fact that type II diabetes is probably a heterogeneous disease, any protein involved in insulin actions or secretion is a potential candidate for an alteration genetically linked to the disease.

Molecular Defects of Insulin Receptor

The cloning of the insulin receptor cDNA [2, 3] and gene [4] recently provided the opportunity to investigate potential molecular mutations as the source of insulin resistance. Attention has been focused firstly on genetic extreme insulin resistance syndromes with functional defects of the insulin receptor. Type A insulin resistance, leprechaunism, lipoatrophic diabetes and Rabson-Mendenhall syndromes were the first investigated.

Methodological Problems

Identification of a single nucleotide mutation responsible for an amino acid substitution in the sequence of the insulin receptor of any patient is now possible with the development of the polymerase chain reaction (PCR) technique. The genetic material can be genomic DNA, purified from the leukocytes contained in a blood sample or mRNA isolated either from Epstein-Barr virus (EBV)-transformed leukocytes or from a fibroblast primary culture obtained by skin biopsy, or from any tissue obtained by biopsy. In this genetic material, the sequences coding for the insulin receptor can be specifically amplified by PCR and therefore analyzed. This analysis includes sequencing of the amplified DNA material or dot blot hybridization with wild type or mutated probes, which identifies already described mutation. Genomic DNA is more easily obtained but it is necessary to individually amplify the 22 exons coding for the insulin receptor, whereas cDNA sequences obtained from mRNA of tissues expressing the insulin receptor require a restricted number of PCR amplifications.

Insulin Receptor Mutations in Extreme Insulin Resistance

Approximately 20 different mutations have been identified and are responsible for syndromes of extreme insulin resistance [15–19]. These mutations are almost uniformly distributed throughout the insulin receptor sequence (fig. 2). Missense mutations represent 12 different cases, whereas 5 families present a nonsense mutation and one a large deletion of the β subunit C-terminal part.

No correlation can be clearly observed between the location of the mutation and the nature of the insulin resistance syndrome. Leprechaunism is exclusively associated with mutations of the extracellular part of the insulin receptor, but type A insulin resistance and Rabson-

Mendenhall syndromes are associated with an equal number of extracellular and intracellular mutations. These mutations are associated with different types of insulin receptor defects, including decrease of mRNA levels, reduction of insulin receptor transport to the cell membrane, modifications of the binding properties and tyrosine kinase defects. In many cases, the location of the mutation explains logically the nature of the defect: all the modifications of insulin binding are due to mutations of the extracellular domain and all the tyrosine kinase alterations are due to mutations in the tyrosine kinase domain. However, in some cases the relationship is not straightforward: nonsense mutations determine essentially a decrease of the mRNA levels or sometimes a defect in the receptor transport. It is also interesting to compare the location of these natural mutations with the sequences identified in parallel by in vitro site-directed mutagenesis as important for the receptor functions. These in vitro studies have already identified short sequences essential for insulin binding (Phe88 to Phe89 and Cys241 to Trp251), subunit cleavage (Arg732 to Arg735), endocytosis (Gln956 to Asp977), tyrosine kinase activity (Gly1003 to Lys1030, Asp1132 to Asn1137 and Pro1172 to Glu1179) and for autophosphorylation (Tyr1158 to Tyr1163 and Tyr1328 to Tyr1334). Interestingly enough, only 3 of the 18 natural mutations already identified concern these sequences [15]. This comparison highlights the still very limited knowledge of the insulin receptor structure-function relationship.

Neither the nature or location of the mutation, nor the nature of the insulin receptor defect allow the prediction of the nature of the insulin resistance syndrome. The very different presentation of these syndromes suggests that other genetic defects are probably associated with some of them. No mutation of the insulin receptor has been described for or associated with lipoatrophic diabetes, which suggests that this syndrome is probably not due to genetic alteration of this receptor.

Finally, the major insulin receptor defects observed in leprechaunism or type A insulin resistance seem to be inconsistent with the presence of a mutation on a single allele of the gene, since the normal gene should produce 50% of normal insulin receptors. In fact, 50% of the familial cases already studied for these mutations present mutations on both genes, being either homozygous for the mutation (3 cases) or compound heterozygotes (5 cases). The others are thought to be simple heterozygotes, but the other allele has not always been completely sequenced, opening the possibility of another mutation. However, the recent demonstration that nonfunctional mutants of the insulin receptor, when expressed at the cell surface, inhibit the normal receptors by forming nonfunctional hybrids [20], may explain the dominant effect of a single gene mutation.

Insulin Receptor Mutations and Type II Diabetes

Mutations or genetic alterations of the insulin receptor are one of the hypotheses which may explain the insulin resistance observed during type II diabetes. The reversibility of the receptor alterations, such as their reduced number at the cell surface, during the treatment or when cells are incubated in vitro, did not completely exclude the fact that a molecular defect of the action of insulin is responsible for the disease in some families. Therefore, the cloning of the insulin receptor offered a new tool to investigate this theory. A genetic linkage between the type II diabetes (phenotype) and some alleles of the insulin receptor gene, identified by restriction fragment length polymorphism (RFLP) (genotype), was investigated in the diabetic population or families [21, 22]. Contradictory results did not allow a clear-cut answer concerning this linkage. This could be due to the heterogeneity of the type II diabetic population or to an absence of direct involvement of the insulin receptor in this syndrome. The later possibility is sustained by the absence of mutation of the insulin receptor gene detected in some familial type II diabetic patients [23] and in the Pima Indians [24], who present a familial and genetically determined type II diabetes. A recent study, analyzing the nature of the insulin receptor subtypes expressed in the muscle of type II diabetic patients as compared to nondiabetic controls, seems to indicate however an abnormal regulation of the insulin receptor gene during diabetes. The presence of the subtype B (low affinity) in the muscle of the 10 diabetic patients, whereas only subtype A was observed in the controls, should be confirmed in a large number of patients, but is an interesting observation [25]. The genetic or acquired nature of this modification and its relationship with insulin resistance should be studied more precisely.

Postreceptor Alterations

Despite the large number of proteins involved in the very complex signalling pathways, which determine the actions of insulin, a restricted number of studies were performed to identify molecular alterations of postreceptor steps. These investigations concern only the glucose transporters and more recently the glucokinase.

Glucose Transporters

Major progress in the structure and functions of the glucose transporters has been made in recent years [10]. The general structure of these membrane-bound proteins is composed of 12 hydrophobic segments, probably representing membrane-spanning domains. Many different genes code for these transporters in different tissues and at the present time 5 facilitative glucose transporters and a sodium-dependent glucose transporter have been identified (GLUT 1–5 and SGLT1). If molecular defects of some of these transporters have already been identified, none of them give an insulin resistance, since only GLUT4 is functionally dependent of insulin. The mechanism of GLUT4 activation by insulin has been elucidated and involves the translocation of GLUT4 from an intracellular pool to the plasma membrane. A stimulation of GLUT4 gene transcription and of GLUT4 activity are also two possible mechanisms of insulin action.

Mutations of GLUT4 gene are potential sources of insulin resistance, but until now such an association has not been demonstrated. A clear reduction of GLUT4 mRNA levels is observed in the muscle and adipose tissue of type II diabetes and obese patients [26]. This modification is probably secondary to other factors, since no polymorphism or mutation of GLUT4 gene has been observed in such patients, except in 1 diabetic patient presenting a Val383 to Ile point mutation [27]. At the present time, the frequency, the consequence and the relationship of this mutation with insulin resistance are not known.

Glucokinase

Glucokinase in the enzyme involved in the phosphorylation of glucose in glucose-6-phosphate. Its activity is regulated by insulin in the liver, but also in the pancreatic β cells and therefore it can be involved in both insulin secretion and resistance. The human gene was recently cloned, offering the possibility to investigate a genetic linkage between this gene and diseases of glucose homeostasis. Interestingly enough a close linkage was observed in some families presenting a young onset type II diabetes (MODY) [28]. Mutations of the glucokinase gene in these families of a particular form of diabetes is believed to be the cause of the disease. This observation opens a new avenue to investigate the molecular alterations responsible for type II diabetes.

Conclusion

The identification of the genetic defects responsible for insulin resistance benefits largely from the development of the tools of recombinant DNA technology. These tools have already attributed the extreme insulin resistance observed in type A insulin resistance and leprechaunism to mutations of the insulin receptor gene. Logically, the future developments of these investigations should concentrate on the molecular alterations responsible for post-receptor insulin resistance. Preliminary results concerning glucose transporters and glucokinase are promising, but a better knowledge of the intracellular mechanisms of insulin action is essential to answer this question. These investigations should also be applied to type II diabetes in order to clarify the involvement of insulin resistance in the pathogenesis of this disease and to elucidate if this syndrome is due to a unique cause or multiple factors.

References

1 Bell GI, Swain WF, Pictet R, Cordell B, Goodman HM, Rutter WJ: Nucleotide sequence of a cDNA clone encoding human preproinsulin. Nature 1979;282:525–527.

2 Ebina Y, Ellis L, Jarnagin K, Edery M, Graf L, Clauser E, Ou J, Masiarz F, Kan YW, Goldfine ID, Roth RA, Rutter WJ: The human insulin receptor cDNA: The structural basis for hormone-activated transmembrane signalling. Cell 1985;40:747–758.

3 Ullrich A, Bell JR, Chen EY, Herrera R, Petruzelli LM, Dull TJ, Gray A, Coussens L, Liao YC, Tsubokawa M, Mason A, Seeburg PH, Grunfeld C, Rosen OM, Ramachandran J: Human insulin receptor and its relationships to the tyrosine kinase family of oncogenes. Nature 1985;313:756–761.

4 Seino S, Seino M, Nishi S, Bell GI: Structure of the insulin receptor gene and characterization of its promoter. Proc Natl Acad Sci USA 1989; 86:114–118.

5 Mosthaf L, Grako K, Dull TJ, Coussens L, Ullrich A, McClain DA: Functionally distinct insulin receptors generated by tissue-specific alternative splicing. EMBO J 1990;9:2409–2413.

6 Sale GJ, Smith DM: Serine phosphorylations triggered by the insulin receptor. Cell Signal 1989;1:205–218.

7 Rosen OM: After insulin binds. Science 1987; 237:1452–1458.

8 Low MG, Saltiel AR: Structural and functional roles in glycosylphosphatidylinositol in membranes. Science 1988;239:268–275.

9 Girard J, Ferre P: Mécanismes d'action cellulaire de l'insuline; in Tchobroutsky G, Slama G, Assan R, Freychet P (eds): Traité de Diabétologie. Paris, Pradel, 1990, pp 141–149.

10 Burant CF, Sivitz WI, Fukumoto H, Kayano T, Nagamatsu S, Seino S, Pessin JE, Bell GI: Mammalian glucose transporters: Structure and molecular regulation. Recent Prog Horm Res 1991;47:349–388.
11 Kahn CR: The molecular mechanism of insulin action. Annu Rev Med 1985;36:429–451.
12 Canivet B, Freychet P: Syndromes d'insulino-résistance extrême et insulinopathies; in Tchobroutsky G, Slama G, Assan R, Freychet P (eds): Traité de Diabétologie. Paris, Pradel, 1990, pp 383–390.
13 Kahn CR, Flier JS, Bar RS, Archer JA, Gorden P, Martin MM, Roth J: The syndromes of insulin resistance and acanthosis nigricans. N Engl J Med 1976;294:739–745.
14 Flier JS: Insulin receptors and insulin resistance. Annu Rev Med 1983;34:145–160.
15 Taylor SI, Kadowaki T, Accili D, Cama A, Kadowaki H, McKeon C, Moncada V, Marcus Samuels B, Bevins C, Ojamaa K, Frapier C, Beitz L, Perrotti N, Rees-Jones R, Margolis R, Imano E, Najjar S, Courtney F, Arakaki R, Gorden R, Roth J: Mutations in the insulin receptor gene in genetic forms of insulin resistance. Recent Prog Horm Res 1990;46:185–217.
16 Moller DE, Yokota A, White MF, Pazianos AG, Flier JS: A naturally occurring mutation of insulin receptor alanine-1134 impairs tyrosine kinase function and is associated with dominantly inherited insulin resistance. J Biol Chem 1990;265:14979–14985.
17 Kusari J, Takata Y, Hatada E, Freidenberg G, Kolterman O, Olefsky JM: Insulin resistance and diabetes due to different mutations in the tyrosine kinase domain of both insulin receptor gene alleles. J Biol Chem 1991;266:5260–5267.
18 Shimada F, Taira M, Suzuki Y, Hashimoto N, Nozaki O, Taira M, Tatibana M, Ebina Y, Tawata M, Onaya T: Insulin-resistant diabetes associated with partial deletion of insulin-receptor gene. Lancet 1990;335:1179–1181.
19 Van der Vorm ER, Van der Zon GC, Moller W, Krans HM, Lindhout D, Maassen JA: An Arg for Gly substitution at position 31 in the insulin receptor, linked to insulin resistance, inhibits receptor processing and transport. J Biol Chem 1992;267:66–71.
20 Treadway JL, Morrison BD, Soos MA, Siddle K, Olefsky J, Ullrich A, McClain DA, Pessin JE: Transdominant inhibition of tyrosine kinase activity in mutant insulin/insulin-like growth factor-I hybrid receptors. Proc Natl Acad Sci USA 1991;88:214–218.
21 McClain DA, Henry RR, Ullrich A, Olefsky JM: Restriction-fragment-length polymorphism in insulin-receptor gene and insulin resistance in NIDDM. Diabetes 1988;37:1071–1075.
22 Morgan R, Bishop A, Owens DR, Luzio SD, Peters JR, Rees A: Allelic variants at insulin-receptor and insulin gene loci and susceptibility to NIDDM in Welsh population. Diabetes 1990;39:1479–1484.
23 Kusari J, Olefsky JM, Strahl C, McClain DA: Insulin-receptor cDNA sequence in NIDDM patient homozygous for insulin-receptor gene RFLP. Diabetes 1991;40:249–254.
24 Moller DE, Yokota A, Flier JS: Normal insulin-receptor cDNA sequence in Pima Indians with NIDDM. Diabetes 1989;38:1496–1500.
25 Mosthaf L, Vogt B, Haring HU, Ullrich A: Altered expression of insulin receptor type-A and type-B in the skeletal muscle of non-insulin-dependent diabetes mellitus patients. Proc Natl Acad Sci USA 1991;88:4728–4730.
26 Garvey WT, Maianu L, Huecksteadt TP, Birnbaum MJ, Molina JM, Ciaraldi TP: Pretranslational suppression of a glucose transporter protein causes insulin resistance in adipocytes from patients with non-insulin-dependent diabetes mellitus and obesity. J Clin Invest 1991;87:1072–1081.
27 Kusari J, Verma US, Buse JB, Henry RR, Olefsky JM: Analysis of the gene sequences of the insulin receptor and the insulin-sensitive glucose transporter (GLUT-4) in patients with common-type non-insulin-dependent diabetes mellitus. J Clin Invest 1991;88:1323–1330.
28 Froguel P, Vaxillaire M, Sun F, Vehlo G, Zouali H, Butel MO, Lesage S, Vionnet N, Clement K, Fougerousse F, Tanizawa Y, Weissenbach J, Beckmann JS, Lathrop GM, Passa P, Permutt MA, Cohen D: Close linkage of glucokinase on chromosome 7p to early-onset non-insulin-dependent diabetes mellitus. Nature 1992;356:162–164.

Horm Res 1992;38:13–18

Jean-Louis Carpentier

Department of Morphology,
University of Geneva Medical Center,
Geneva, Switzerland

Insulin-Induced and Constitutive Internalization of the Insulin Receptor

Key Words
Insulin receptor
Endocytosis

Abstract

The characterization of the cellular and molecular mechanisms governing insulin receptor internalization is of crucial importance to better define the functional role of this process in insulin receptor regulation and insulin action both in normal and pathological conditions.

In the present work we have characterized the factors intrinsic to the receptor which are responsible for the triggering and regulation of insulin receptor internalization. We found that: (a) insulin induces the internalization of its receptor via activation of the tyrosine kinase intrinsic to the cytoplasmic domain of the molecule; (b) this ligand-specific step consists in the redistribution of the receptor from microvilli where binding occurs to the nonvillous region of the cell surface where internalization occurs; (c) the second step of the internalization process, i.e. association with clathrin-coated pits, requires a consensus sequence of the juxtamembrane domain of the receptor, and (d) this step is ligand-independent and is responsible for the constitutive internalization of the receptor.

Background

The insulin receptor is an integral plasma membrane glycoprotein which recognizes and binds insulin. It consists of four subunits: two exoplasmic α-subunits are linked by disulfide bonds to two transmembrane β-subunits. Both α and β-subunits are synthesized by way of a single chain proreceptor which is cleaved and further processed prior to insertion into the plasma membrane [1]. The cDNA encoding the proreceptor has been cloned and the protein sequence of the receptor elucidated [2, 3]. Insulin binds to the α-subunit and activates a tyrosine-specific protein kinase intrinsic to the cytoplasmic domain of the β-subunit. The activation of this kinase leads to the autophosphorylation of the receptor on tyrosine residues (fig. 1).

Following its expression on the cell surface the insulin receptor can be removed by receptor-mediated endocytosis (fig. 2). This process involves: (a) the inital interaction of insulin with its receptor on thin digitations of the cell surface: the microvilli; (b) the redistribution of the insulin-receptor complex in the plane of the membrane and the concentration of this complex in clathrin-coated pits which pinch off to form clathrin-coated vesicles; (c) the internalization of the insulin-receptor complex; (d) the dissociation of insulin from its receptor in endosomes and

Jean-Louis Carpentier
Department of Morphology
University of Geneva Medical Center
1, rue Michel-Servet
CH–1211 Geneva 4 (Switzerland)

0301–0163/92/0382–0013
$2.75/0

1

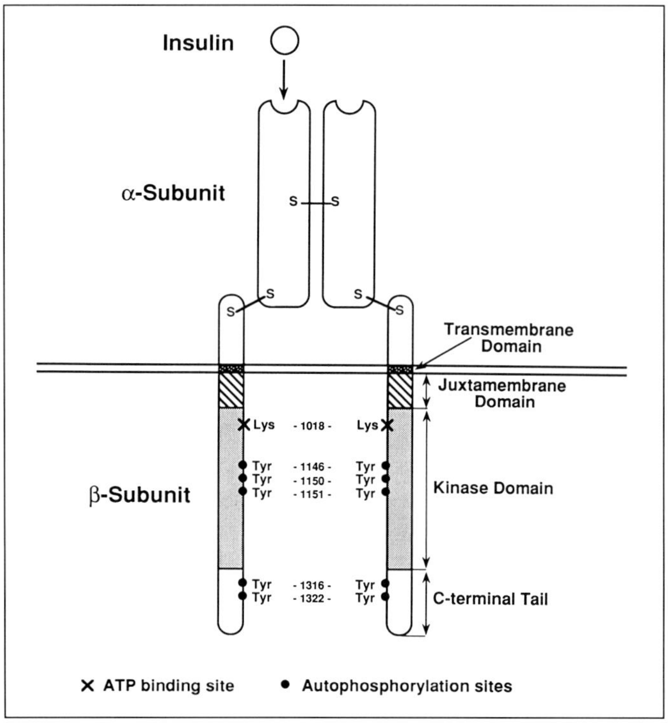

2

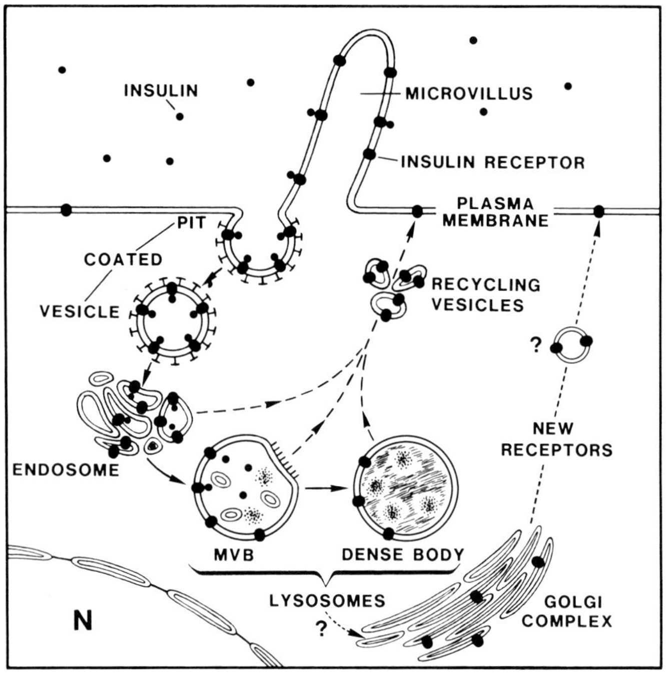

Fig. 1. Schematic view of the insulin receptor with its two external binding domains (α-subunits) linked by disulfide bonds to two transmembrane domains (β-subunits) extending into the cytoplasm. The cytoplasmic segment of the β-subunit includes a juxtamembrane domain, the kinase domain and the C-terminal tail. Following insulin binding to the α-subunit the receptor becomes phosphorylated on specific tyrosine residue.

Fig. 2. Schematic representation of the surface localization and intracellular pathway of insulin and its receptor [from 4].

its subsequent degradation in endosomes and lysosomes, and (e) the recycling of the insulin receptor back to the cell surface [4].

Internalization of the insulin-receptor complexes plays a key role in the regulation and control of the biological action of the hormone by allowing the intracellular degradation of insulin and the modulation of the number of surface insulin receptors [4–8]. This is true not only in normal but also in pathological conditions: for example, in two situations of decreased extracellular insulin level, streptozotocin diabetes in rats and type I (insulin-dependent) diabetes mellitus in man, we observed a significantly reduced internalization rate of insulin, this reduction was corrected by insulin treatment [9]. In monocytes of type II diabetic patients and of lipoatrophic diabetic patients, ^{125}I-insulin internalization was also decreased [10]; in these conditions an intrinsic defect in the mechanism of internalization is probably present and could be responsible for the altered biological response to the hormone.

Endocytosis of the insulin receptor is triggered by insulin binding [4, 6,11] but the mechanism underlying this process remains unclear. Since insulin-receptor internalization required energy, it was recently proposed that kinase activation and receptor autophosphorylation were implicated in this process. Unfortunately, at present, data collected on this subject are controversial [12–18]. Moreover, other domains of the cytoplasmic segment of the β-subunit of the insulin receptor could also be implicated in the internalization process. The juxtamembrane domain, including a consensus sequence involved in internalization of various receptors, seems required for insulin-receptor endocytosis [19–23]. The C-terminal tail of the β-subunit could also play a role in internalization and could represent a regulatory domain as described in the case of the EGF receptor [24].

The aim of the present work was to distinguish which receptor domains are implicated in the various steps of the internalization process. To this end, we have tracked directly, by quantitative electron microscopy (EM) autoradiography, ^{125}I-insulin [25–27] on the surface and inside cells transfected with normal human insulin receptors or insulin receptors with mutations selected to provide information about the role of the various domains of the β-subunit. Results summarized in this review have been presented in detail in previous papers [27, 28].

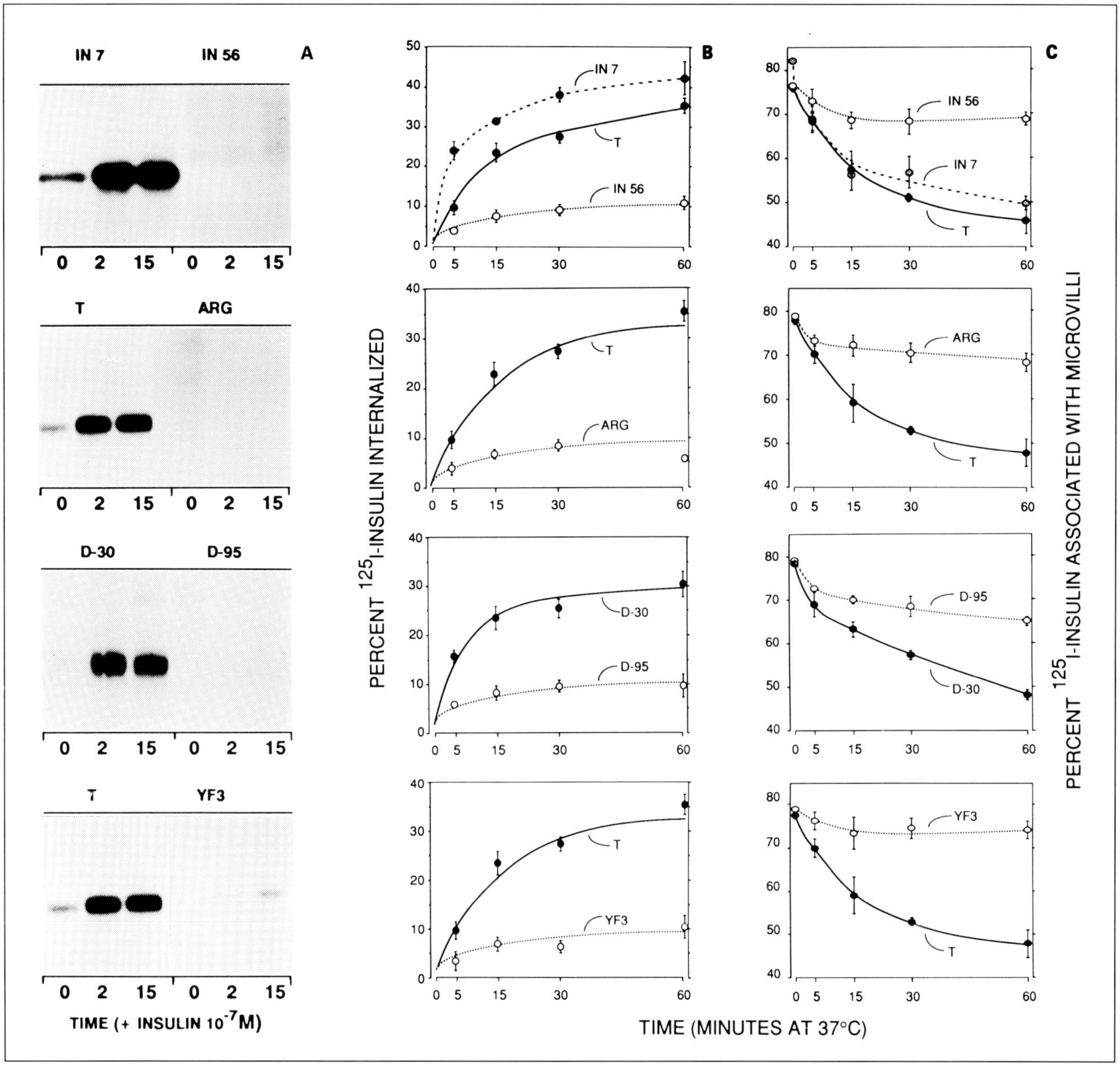

Fig. 3. A Insulin-induced phosphorylation of its receptor in the various CHO cells. **B** ^{125}I-insulin internalization. **C** Surface redistribution from microvilli to the nonvillous surface in the various CHO cells under study [adapted from 27].

Results and Discussion

First, we have studied the implication of the intrinsic kinase activity of the receptor in its insulin-induced internalization. To that end, we have followed ^{125}I-insulin by quantitative EM autoradiography as previously described [30, 31]. The internalization process was studied in a battery of CHO cells transfected either with normal human insulin receptors or human insulin receptors mutated so as to affect kinase activation. The following mutations (prepared by Dr. W.J. Rutter, University of California, San Francisco, Calif.) were studied: replacement of the

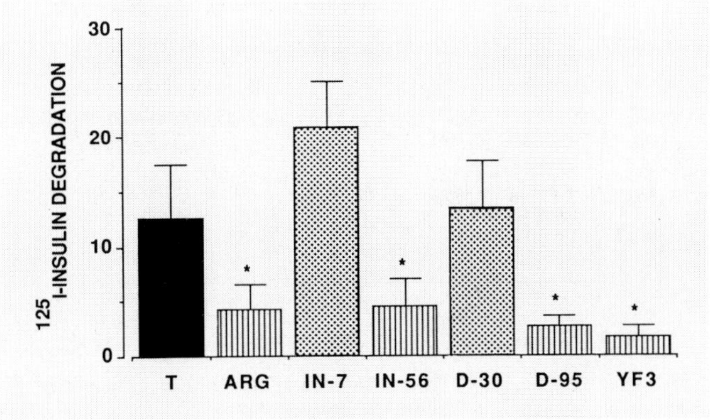

Fig. 4. ^{125}I-insulin degradation by the various CHO cell lines under study [From 27].

lysine residue at 1018 by arginine (CHO.ARG) [16]: truncation of 95 COOH-terminal amino acids (CHO.D-95) [16]; juxamembrane insertions obtained by multimerization of residues 946–952 (one time the 7 amino acid spacers = CHO.IN-7; eight times the same spacer = CHO.IN-56) [29].

Phosphorylation of the human insulin receptor of CHO.T and CHO.IN-7 cell lines was stimulated by insulin (fig. 3). By contrast, CHO.IN-56, CHO.ARG, and CHO.D-95 exhibited completely inhibited insulin-dependent phosphorylation.

CHO.T cells progressively internalized ^{125}I-insulin so that by 60 min of incubation, 35–40% of the cell-associated radioactive material was inside the cells (fig. 3). Similar results were obtained with CHO.IN-7 cells, except that in this case, the internalization was slightly increased (fig. 3). By contrast, ^{125}I-insulin internalization was inhibited in the 3 CHO cell lines transfected with insulin receptors with mutations affecting the kinase activity (fig. 3). Since insulin degradation depends upon receptor-mediated endocytosis [4], we have assessed the degradation of ^{125}I-insulin in the incubation medium of the various CHO cells at the end of 60 min incubation period at 37 °C. The level of ^{125}I-insulin degradation was markedly reduced in CHO.ARG, IN-56, and D-95 cells as compared to the one observed in CHO.T, IN-7, and D-30 cells (fig. 4). Thus ^{125}I-insulin internalization and degradation are strongly correlated with receptor kinase activation.

In the second part of this work we tried to determine whether an intact kinase was sufficient or whether, in addition, autophosphorylation of specific tyrosine residues of the receptor was required for insulin to induce internalization of its receptor. To that end, we followed ^{125}I-insulin internalization in cells expressing insulin receptors with deletion or substitution of the major sites of autophosphorylation. Deletion of 30 amino acids of the β-subunit (CHO.D-30) which removed two autophosphorylation sites (1316 and 1322) but maintained a normal kinase activity was without effect on ^{125}I-insulin internalization (fig. 3). By contrast, substitution of the two tyrosines of the kinase or regulatory domain (1150 and 1151) for phenylalanine [30] resulted in an inhibition of ^{125}I-insulin internalization in spite of the fact that the insulin receptor kinase was activated (fig. 3). Thus, insulin receptor internalization requires not only an intact and activable kinase but also the autophosphorylation of specific tyrosine residues.

The extent of internalization of polypeptide hormone is correlated with their degree of lateral mobility [31]. To determine whether autophosphorylation is required for insulin-induced surface redistribution of the receptor, we localized ^{125}I-insulin on the surface of the various CHO cells. With incubation time at 37 °C, ^{125}I-insulin shifted from microvilli to nonvillous domains in all cell lines with normal kinase activity and preserved autophosphorylation sites in the regulatory domain of the molecule (fig.3). By contrast, in kinase-inactive and/or autophosphorylation-deficient cells, ^{125}I-insulin redistribution was inhibited (fig. 3). Thus, kinase activation and autophosphorylation (especially of tyrosine residues 1150 and 1151) of the insulin receptor provides a mechanism by which insulin triggers the ligand-specific step of receptor internalization, i.e. the surface redistribution of the receptor from microvilli to the nonvillous surface of the cells.

The second step of the internalization process appears more general and common to many receptors, including those which are not autophosphorylated: it consists in the anchoring of the receptor in clathrin-coated pits. This step may involve specific amino acid sequences which have been found in the cytoplasmic tail of many receptors [19]. Preliminary results indicate that this step requires the presence of a preserved juxtamembrane domain including a GPLY and an NPXY sequence and that exposed aromatic residues in positions 953 and 960 are crucial for association with clathrin-coated pits and internalization [20, 22, 23].

But even in the absence of kinase activation, a small percentage of ^{125}I-insulin enters the cells (fig. 3). To trace this insulin-independent pathway of internalization, we followed by quantitative EM autoradiography a monoclonal antibody directed against the α-subunit of the human insulin receptor (mAb 83-14). The internalization of this antibody was comparable in CHO cells expressing kinase-active or kinase-inactive receptors and was similar to that observed for ^{125}I-insulin in kinase-inactive cells. Thus this antibody which does not activate insulin receptor kinase at the concentration used is an appropriate tool to study the constitutive internalization of the insulin receptor.

As shown morphologically, ^{125}I-mAb-83-14 present on the nonvillous region of the cells, where internalization occurs, preferentially associated with clathrin-coated pits, which demonstrates that these surface invaginations are not only implicated in insulin-induced but also constitutive internalization of the insulin receptor [28].

The data that we have reviewed indicate that insulin binds to a specific cell surface receptor. The complex then becomes involved in a series of steps which lead the insulin-receptor complex to be internalized and rapidly dissociated: the hormone is degraded in lysosomes and the receptor is recycled back to the cell surface. This sequence of events participates in the regulation of the cell sensitivity to the hormone both in normal and pathological conditions. Except for the first step of internalization (surface redistribution), the sequence of events closely resembles what is observed in the case of many unrelated ligands such as low density lipoproteins, toxins, lectins and viruses. Thus, one can distinguish two degrees of specificity in the course of the internalization of the insulin receptor: first a ligand-dependent step which requires insulin-induced receptor phosphorylation of specific tyrosine residues and allows the receptor to leave microvilli where it preferentially localizes in its unoccupied form, and second a more general step common to many other receptors: the association with clathrin-coated pits which represent the internalization gate common to many receptors.

Acknowledgments

This work has been supported by grant 31-34093.92 from the Swiss National Science Foundation, the Juvenile Diabetes Foundation and a grant-in-aid-from NOVO Baegsvaerd, Denmark.

References

1 Hedo JA, Kahn CR, Hayashi M, Yamada KM, Kasuga M: Biosynthesis and glycosylation of the insulin receptor. Evidence for a single polypeptide precursor of the two major subunits. J. Biol Chem 1983;258:10020–10026.

2 Ebina Y, Ellis L, Jarnagin K, Edery M, Graf L, Clauser E, Ou JH, Masiarz F, Kan YW, Goldfine ID, Roth RA, Rutter WJ: The human insulin receptor cDNA: The structural basis for hormone-activated transmembrane signalling. Cell 1985;40:747 758.

3 Ullrich A, Bell JR, Chen EY, Herrera R, Petruzzelli LM, Dull TJ, Gray A, Coussens L, Liao YC, Tsubokawa M, Mason A, Seeburg PH, Grunfeld C, Rosen OM, Ramanchandran J: Human insulin receptor and its relationship to the tyrosine kinase family of oncogenes. Nature 1985;313:756–761.

4 Carpentier JL: The cell biology of the insulin receptor. Diabetologia 1989;32:627–635.

5 Gorden P, Freychet P, Carpentier JL, Canivet B, Orci L: Receptor linked degradation of ^{125}I-insulin is mediated by inernalization in isolated rat hepatocytes. Yale J Biol Med 1982;55: 101–112.

6 Carpentier JL, Dayer JM, Lang U, Silverman R, Orci L, Gorden P: Down-regulation and recycling of insulin receptors: Effects of monensin on IM-lymphocytes and U-937 monocyte-type cells. J Biol Chem 1984;259:14180–14195.

7 Geiger D, Carpentier JL, Gorden P, Orci L: Down-regulation of insulin receptors is related to insulin internalization. Exp Cell Res 1989; 185:33–40.

8 Gorden P, Carpentier JL, Freychet P, Orci L: Internalization of polypeptide hormones. Mechanism, intracellular localization and significance. Diabetologia 1980;18:263–274.

9 Carpentier JL, Robert A, Grunberger G, Van Obberghen E, Freychet P, Orci L, Gorden P: Receptor-mediated endocytosis of polypeptide hormones is a regulated process: Inhibition of [^{125}I] iodoinsulin internalization in hypoinsulinemic diabetes of rat and man. J Clin Endocrinol Metab 1986;63:151–155.

10 Grunberger G, Geiger D, Carpentier JL, Robert A, Gorden P: Receptor-mediated endocytosis of insulin. Inhibition of [^{125}I]iodoinsulin internalization in insulin resistant diabetic staes of man. Acta Endocrinol (Copenh) 1989; 121:581–586.

11 Backer JM, Kahn CR, White MF: Tyrosine phosphorylation of the insulin receptor during insulin-stimulated internalization in rat hepatoma cells. J Biol Chem 1989;264:1694–1701.

12 Hari J, Roth RA: Defective internalization of insulin and its receptor in cells expressing mutated insulin receptors lacking kinase activity. J Biol Chem 1987;262:15341–15344.

13 McClain DA, Maegawa H, Lee J, Dull TJ, Ullrich A, Olefsky JM: A mutant insulin receptor with defective tyrosine kinase displays no biologic activity and does not undergo endocytosis. J Biol Chem 1987;262:14663–14671.

14 Russel DS, Gherzi R, Johnson El, Chou CK, Rosen O: The protein-tyrosine kinase activity of the insulin receptor is necessary for insulin-mediated receptor down-regulation. J Biol Chem 1987;262:11833–11840.

15 Reynet C, Caron M, Magre GC, Clauser E, Picard J, Capeau J: Mutation of tyrosine residues 1162 and 1163 of the insulin receptor affects hormone and receptor internalization. Mol Endocrinol 1990;4:304–311.

16 Berhanu P, Rohilla A, Brandeburg D, Aggerberk M: A deletion mutation of the human insulin receptor causing loss of kinase activity does not impair internalization and processing (abstract). Diabetes 1988;37:(suppl):2A.

17 Backer JM, Kahn CR, White MF: Tyrosine phosphorylation of the insulin receptor internalization studies with 2,4-dinitrophenol-treated cells. Proc Natl Acad Sci USA 1989;86: 3209–3213.

18 Trischitta V, Wong KY, Brunetti A, Scalisi R, Vigneri R, Goldfine ID: Endocytosis, recycling, and degradation of the insulin receptor. J Biol Chem 1989;264:5041–5046.

19 Chen WJ, Goldstein JL, Brown MS: NPXY, a sequence often found in cytoplasmic tail, is required for coated pit-mediated internalization of the low density lipoprotein receptor. J Biol Chem 1990;265:3116–3123.

20 Thies RS, Webster NJ, McClain DA: A domain of the insulin receptor required for endocytosis in rat fibroblasts. J Biol Chem 1990;265: 10132–10137.

21 Backer JM, Shoelson SE, Weiss MA, Hua QX, Cheatham RB, Haring E, Cahill DC, White MF: The insulin receptor juxtamembrane region contains two independent tyrosine/β-turn internalization signals. J Cell Biol 1992;118: 831–839.
22 Backer JM, Kahn CR, Cahill DA, Ullrich A, White MF: Receptor-mediated internalization of insulin requires a 12-amino acid sequence in the juxtamembrane region of the insulin receptor beta subunit. J Biol Chem 1990;265: 16450–16454.
23 Rajagopalan M, Neidigh JL, McClain DA: Amino acid sequences Gly-Pro-Leu-Tyr and Asn-Pro-Glu-Tyr in the submembranous domain of the insulin recptor are required for normal endocytosis. J Biol Chem 1991;266: 23068–23073.
24 Chen MS, Lazar CS, Lund KA, Welsh JB, Chang C, Walton CM, Der CJ, Wiley HJ, Gill GN, Rosenfeld MG: Functional independence of the epidermal growth factor receptor from a domain required for ligand-induced internalization and calcium regulation. Cell 1989;59: 33–43.
25 Carpentier JL, Gorden P, Amherdt M, Van Obberghen E, Kahn CR, Orci L: ^{125}I-insulin binding to cultured human lymphocytes. Initial localization and fate of hormone determined by quantitative electron microscope autoradiography. J Clin Invest 1978;61:1057–1070.
26 Carpentier JL, Gorden O, Anderson RGW, Goldstein JL, Brown MS, Cohen S, Orci L: Colocalization of ^{125}I-epidermal growth factor and ferritin-low density lipoprotein in coated pits: A quantitative electron microscopic study in normal and mutant human fibroblasts. J Cell Biol 1982;95:73–77.
27 Carpentier JL, Paccaud JP, Gorden P, Rutter WJ, Orci L: Insulin-induced surface redistribution regulates internalization of the insulin receptor and requires its autophosphorylation. Proc Natl Sci USA 1992;89:162–166.
28 Paccaud JP, Siddle K, Carpentier JL: Internalization of the human insulin receptor. J Biol Chem 1992;18:13101–13106.
29 Rohilla A, Bertanu P, Furukawa H, Rutter WJ: Insertional mutations in the peri-membranous region of the human insulin receptor intracytoplasmic domain perturb its internalization. Diabetes 1989;(suppl 2):60A.
30 Ellis L, Clauser E, Morgan DO, Edery M, Roth RA, Rutter WJ: Replacement of insulin receptor tyrosine residues 1162 and 1163 compromises insulin-stimulated kinase activity and uptake of 2-deoxyglucose. Cell 1986;45:721–732.
31 De Diego JG, Gorden P, Carpentier JL: The relationship of ligand receptor mobility with the internalization of polypeptide hormones and growth factors. Endocrinology 1991;128: 2136–2140.

Horm Res 1992;38:19–27

A.J. Scheen
P.J. Lefèbvre

Division of Diabetes, Nutrition and Metabolic Disorders, Department of Medicine, CHU Liège, Sart Tilman, Liège, Belgium

Assessment of Insulin Resistance in vivo: Application to the Study of Type 2 Diabetes

Key Words
Glucose clamp
Glucose kinetics
Insulin resistance
Insulin secretion
Insulin sensitivity
Intravenous glucose tolerance test
Minimal model
Type 2 (noninsulin-dependent) diabetes

Abstract
Besides insulin secretion, insulin sensitivity plays a key role in the feedback glucose-insulin closed loop. It can be altered in numerous physiological, pathological and pharmacological conditions. It can be estimated in vivo using methods that open the feedback loop (insulin suppression test, glucose clamp) or that analyze the closed loop by employing mathematical models of glucose kinetics. The most popular method is the euglycemic hyperinsulinemic glucose clamp. This test should be ideally coupled with a priming-constant infusion of a glucose tracer together with indirect calorimetry. This combination allows to study the glucose kinetics (R_a and R_d, and thus endogenous – mainly hepatic – glucose production) and its metabolism (oxidation or storage as glycogen), respectively. One alternative approach is the frequently sampled intravenous glucose tolerance test where the dynamic changes in plasma insulin and glucose levels are analyzed using the so-called 'minimal model' method. Noninsulin-dependent or type 2 diabetes is characterized by a significant defect in both insulin secretion and action. The insulin resistance is located at the liver site (increased glucose production) and at the peripheral tissues (decreased oxidation and, even more, defective storage of glucose in the muscles). This insulin resistance, which predominates at the postreceptor level, seems to be genetically determined but is worsened by weight excess and by hyperglycemia itself. This contributes to a vicious circle which aggravates progressively the severity of the disease.

Introduction

Insulin sensitivity plays a key role in the glucose-insulin feedback closed loop. There is permanent intercommunication between the insulin-sensitive tissues and the B cells of the pancreas. Variations in glucose production or utilization induce a rapid B-cell secretory compensation in order to maintain normoglycemia; conversely, changes in insulin secretion are quickly reflected in the plasma glucose concentration [1].

For insulin to exert its biological effects, it must be secreted from the islets' B cells, pass through the liver

A.J. Scheen
Division of Diabetes, Nutrition and Metabolic Disorders
Department of Medicine
CHU Liège, Sart Tilman
B–4000 Liège 1 (Belgium)

0301–0163/92/0382–0019
$2.75/0

where it exerts some of its effects, diffuse from the circulation to the interstitium and, finally, reach its target tissues intact. The insulin molecule must then interact with its receptor at the plasma membrane, and this event initiates intracellular processes, resulting in the biological response to the hormone. Any abnormality in this sequence will result in a subnormal response to insulin. This decreased insulin action is called insulin resistance [2, 3].

Insulin resistance plays a significant role in numerous physiological, pathological and pharmacological conditions [2, 4, 5]. For instance, it is present during puberty, pregnancy and in the elderly; it is of importance not only in obesity and diabetes but also in essential hypertension, dyslipidemia and atherosclerotic cardiovascular disease, and finally it is aggravated by various drugs such as glucocorticoids, some contraceptive pills or diuretics, etc.

The purpose of the present review is to describe the main approaches currently used for the evaluation of insulin sensitivity in the intact organism. The application of these techniques in the study of patients with type 2 (noninsulin-dependent) diabetes has markedly increased our knowledge in the pathophysiology of the disease and clearly demonstrated the crucial role played by insulin resistance [4–10].

Measurement of Insulin Resistance in vivo

Historical Background

In the 1930s, Himsworth [11] introduced the first standard approach to measuring insulin sensitivity in vivo. Two oral glucose tolerance tests (OGTT) were performed in individual subjects: one with, and the second without a concomitant intravenous insulin injection. Insulin sensitivity was expressed as the ratio of the areas under the respective glucose tolerance curves. By using this approach, Himsworth showed that young, thin, ketosis-prone (now called type 1) diabetic subjects are more sensitive to exogenous insulin than older, heavier, nonketotic (now called type 2) diabetic patients. Later on, the intravenous insulin tolerance test, without glucose administration, confirmed a blunted decline in plasma glucose concentration in noninsulin-dependent diabetic patients; however, it could expose the subjects to hypoglycemia and thus the results could be artifacted by the counterregulatory response. A similar impairment of insulin action has also been reported using the classical isolated perfused forearm technique [reviewed in 6, 7].

The development of the radioimmunoassay by Yalow and Berson [12] satisfied the need for a sensitive and specific measurement of plasma insulin and allowed an evaluation of insulin sensitivity based upon a quantitative relationship between plasma insulin concentrations and some measurable insulin-dependent metabolic processes. Once this method was validated, various techniques for measuring the in vivo effects of known changes in plasma insulin levels were introduced. For instance, supranormal plasma insulin levels during an OGTT were shown in obese, but nondiabetic, subjects as well as in normal-weight moderately glucose-intolerant subjects [13]. Inappropriately elevated plasma insulin concentrations, in the face of a normal or supranormal plasma glucose pattern during an oral and/or intravenous glucose tolerance test, has come to be accepted as evidence for diminished overall tissue sensitivity to insulin. However, as pointed out by Bergman et al. [14], because of this closed-loop relationship between the B cells of the pancreas and the insulin-sensitive tissues, it is possible only under limited conditions to interpret OGTT results to infer the physiologic status of the extrapancreatic tissues, as of the B cells.

The Open-Loop Approach

A distinct advantage in quantifying insulin sensitivity can be obtained by utilizing methods which prevent the usual feedback relationship between the B cells and the insulin-sensitive tissues [14]. With the feedback loop interrupted, it is possible by exogenous infusion to maintain control over the plasma glucose and/or insulin levels, and to examine the dose-response relationship between insulin and specific metabolic processes. Two distinct classes of methodologies have been applied to open the glucose-insulin feedback relationship in vivo.

The Insulin Suppression Test

One approach, pioneered by Reaven and co-workers [7, 15] and labelled as the pancreatic or insulin suppression test, utilized pharmacological means to render the pancreas blind to the plasma glucose concentration. This could be obtained by infusing epinephrine + propranolol, or somatostatin alone. Insulin is infused to obtain a constant plasma insulin level. Glucose is also infused at a constant rate, and the resultant steady-state plasma glucose (SSPG) concentration is viewed as a measure of the sensitivity of the tissues to insulin. With this technique, Reaven [7] has clearly shown that obese subjects, lean subjects with impaired glucose tolerance, and type 2 diabetic patients uniformly demonstrated the presence of insulin resistance. However, this methodology has been questioned because of several drawbacks: variable effects of the α-adrenergic stimulation (or of the somatostatin administration), nonlinearities in the effects of insulin and glucose on glucose utilization, variable and incomplete suppression of hepatic glucose production, urinary glucose losses, and intervention of the counterregulatory hormones [14]. Consequently, it has been largely supplanted by the glucose clamp technique.

The Glucose Clamp Technique

Of the methods presently available, the euglycemic hyperinsulinemic clamp technique provides the most precise characterization of insulin action on carbohydrate metabolism in vivo. It is an application of the negative feedback principle to the system regulating the plasma glucose level. Andres et al. [16] introduced this technique already in 1966, but it was mainly DeFronzo et al. [17] who were responsible for its monumental exploitation during the last decade, after their remarkable paper published in 1979.

In general, after basal blood sampling, a primed-continuous intravenous infusion of insulin is administered to increase the plasma insulin level to a predetermined concentration. Arterialized blood is sampled at frequent intervals (every 5 min for instance), the glucose concentration is determined immediately, and then a necessary rate of glucose infusion is calculated to attempt to maintain (clamp) plasma glucose at the target value (euglycemia for instance). After an appropriate period, at which steady state is presumed to be reached, the rate of glucose infusion (M) is equal to the rate of peripheral glucose disposal, provided that the plasma insulin levels are high enough to fully suppress endogenous (mainly hepatic) glucose production. M is thus considered an indicator of insulin action at the periphery, mainly the skeletal muscles [17]. When the glucose clamp technique is combined with the isotopic determination of glucose fluxes (using 3-^{3}H-glucose for instance) [18–20], the effects of a specific plasma insulin concentration on individual components of glucose metabolism (production and utilization) can be assessed. The rate of disappearance of glucose (R_d), measured by the isotopic dilution technique, is equivalent to the rate of glucose disposal (a small systematic error could be present when glucose clearance is elevated), while the rate of endogenous glucose production is calculated by subtracting the rate of exogenous glucose infusion M from the total rate of glucose appearance (R_a). Special cautions should be taken to avoid negative values of endogenous

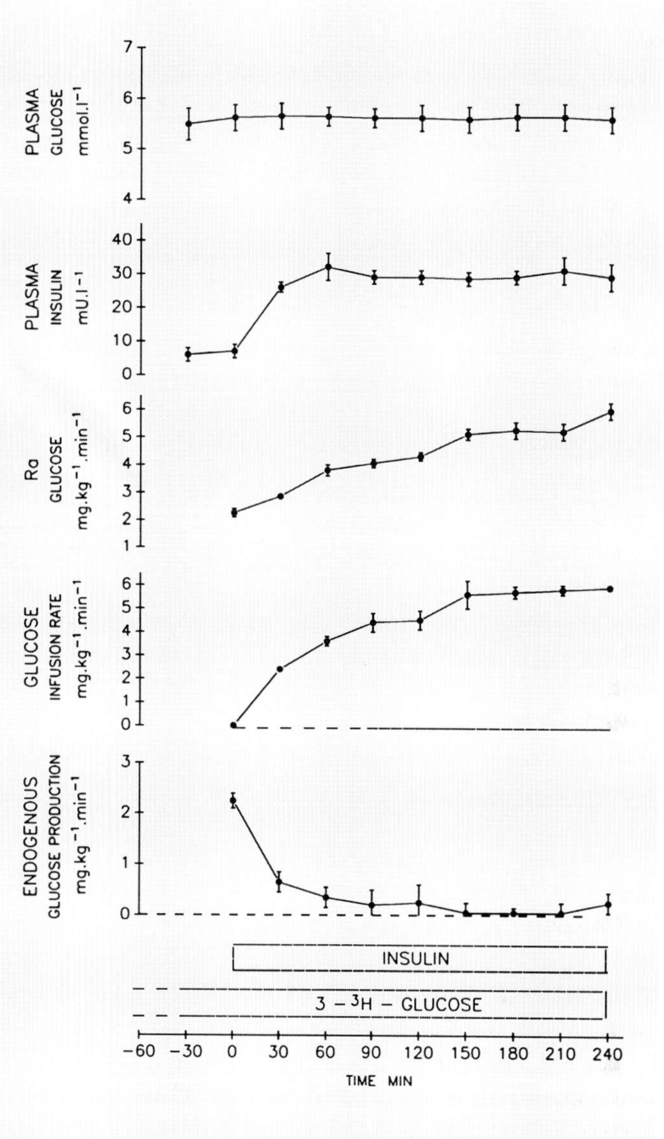

Fig. 1. Illustration of the principle of the euglycemic hyperinsulinemic clamp technique combined with the study of the glucose fluxes using a primed-continuous intravenous infusion of 3-^{3}H-glucose. The results were obtained in 7 healthy young male volunteers connected to an artificial pancreas (Biostator®) and receiving a constant intravenous insulin delivery rate of 0.4 mU·kg^{-1}·min^{-1} from 0 to 240 min. The results are expressed as the mean ± SEM.

glucose production [reviewed in 21]. Figure 1 shows results obtained in normal subjects during a euglycemic hyperinsulinemic clamp combined with the isotopic dilution technique using 3-^{3}H-glucose. The stimulatory effect of insulin on glucose disposal and its inhibitory effect on endogenous glucose production are clearly demonstrated. Moreover, the combination of the glucose clamp with indirect calorimetry allows to measure the fraction of glucose which is oxidized and, by subtracting it from the total amount of infused glucose, the fraction of glucose which is not oxidized and thus considered as stored as glycogen [22–24], providing that there is no significant glycosuria.

Because insulin action may be regulated through changes in insulin receptor binding, Kahn [25] suggested that it would be worthwile to use complete dose-response curves between plasma insulin levels and insulin action in vivo to calculate Michaelis-Menten parameters of insulin action: K_m represents the insulin sensitivity and V_{max} the insulin responsiveness. Classically, a lateral shift of the dose-response curve, leading to a change in the K_m, suggests a change in the binding of insulin to the membrane receptors while a change in the maximal response (V_{max}) suggests a modification in the insulin action beyond the receptor binding process [25, 26]. So, the performance of such a complete dose-response curve in a single individual certainly gives a lot of interesting information, but unfortunately it requires considerable effort and is time-consuming [14, 21].

The development of the glucose clamp was propitious for those interested in measuring insulin sensitivity. This method has the advantage of circumventing most problems discussed above with the insulin suppression test; in particular, the maintenance of euglycemia avoids the difficulties of interpretation of the SSPG and does not require the use of pharmacological agents to suppress endogenous insulin secretion [14, 27]. However, confounding factors still remain [3, 14, 21, 28]: time to reach steady state, glycemia achieved during the clamp (which could be important particularly when comparing subjects with different initial blood glucose levels), nonlinearities in the relationship between glucose, insulin and glucose utilization in the intact organism. The latter are not fully corrected by the use of the metabolic clearance rate (MCR) of glucose (M divided by the steady-state plasma glucose levels), neither by the use of the ratio M/I, i.e. the rate of glucose infusion divided by the steady-state plasma insulin concentrations [3, 14, 21, 28]. Moreover, because of the potential bias inherent to manual control of the glucose infusion rate, a need exists for automatic clamp algorithm using either an artificial pancreas (Biostator®) or a simple mathematical model of glucose regulation implemented on a computer. As a consequence of all these problems, the glucose clamp technique requires skilled staff and is labor-intensive [3, 14, 21, 28].

The Closed-Loop Approach

Some people turn to methods that employ models of glucose kinetics to assess insulin sensitivity with endogenously secreted insulin [28–31]. Evidently these methods are only applicable if there is significant endogenous insulin secretion. By the use of computer modeling, it is possible to circumvent the need to sever the feedback loop between plasma insulin and glucose. This results in protocols which obviate many of the technical complexities inherent in performing the glucose clamp.

Homeostatic Model or Continuous Infusion of Glucose with Model Assessment

In the attempt to simplify the assessment of insulin sensitivity, a 'structural' model may be used, that is one containing the best available physiological data of the normal functions of different organs such as brain, adipose, liver, and skeletal muscle tissues, in order to describe the relationship between glucose and insulin.

In HOMA (Homeostatic Model Assessment) [32], knowing the fasting plasma glucose and insulin levels, it is possible to calculate the insulin sensitivity through the incorporation of physiological data of glucose uptake or production rates by different organs and their known responses to different levels of insulin and glucose. In CIGMA (Continuous Infusion of Glucose with Model Assessment) [33], the endogenous insulin secretion is stimulated by a constant infusion of glucose. The steady-state plasma levels of glucose and insulin are then used to define insulin sensitivity from the model.

However, the major drawback of a structural model is that several variables are not individualized for each subject studied, and such variables could differ in disease [28]. Moreover, in HOMA and CIGMA, the insulin sensitivity is determined from a single pair of values of plasma insulin and glucose, rather than from the dynamics of a whole range of such values.

Frequently Sampled Intravenous Glucose Tolerance Test with Minimal Modeling

This approach to measuring insulin sensitivity uses an intravenous injection of glucose (bolus of $0.3\ g \cdot kg^{-1}$) to stimulate endogenous insulin secretion. Frequent blood samples are collected at intervals over 3 h, for estimation of plasma insulin and glucose levels. If an appropriate model of glucose metabolism can be implemented, and the measured insulin pattern is supplied to it, the computer model may infer individual proper insulin sensitivity in the process of accounting for the measured plasma glucose dynamics [3, 21, 30, 34].

The model has to be simple (or minimal) so that the parameters of glucose metabolism can be identified and individualized for each subject. Yet it has to be complex enough to reflect accurately glucose disposal mechanisms after intravenous glucose injection. The model selected by Bergman et al. [34] assumes that injected glucose is distributed rapidly in a single compartment and that plasma glucose falls by one of two mechanisms: a component that is independent of the incremental insulin response (glucose effectiveness index or S_g) and a component which is dependent on the insulin response, producing an insulin action in an active compartment (insulin sensitivity index or S_i).

Figure 2 illustrates the principle of the minimal model approach and gives preliminary results of the reproducibility of the index of insulin sensitivity S_i in 7 normal subjects submitted to two frequently sampled intravenous tolerance tests (FSIVGTT) 1 week apart. The intrasubject reproducibility of S_i was rather good but the inter-subject variability was rather large within this normal population. These results have to be confirmed in a greater number of subjects.

One disadvantage of the minimal modelling technique is that it is unable to fractionate the insulin-independent and -dependent mechanisms of glucose clearance to hepatic and peripheral components. Clearly, the measure of insulin sensitivity S_i will reflect insulin action at both these sites and isotopic determination is mandatory to discriminate the two effects [28, 35]. Another disadvantage is the need for a large insulin response to obtain an accurate measure of S_i. This requirement leads their promoters to propose an intravenous injection of tolbutamide (or of insulin) 20 min after the glucose administration, particularly in subjects with low glucose-induced insulin secretion such as lean physically active normal subjects and diabetic patients [21, 30].

Several studies have reported a good correlation between the indices of insulin sensitivity measured by the minimal model approach and by the clamp technique [reviewed in 21]. Perhaps the FSIVGTT more closely describes insulin sensitivity in the real life as changes in plasma insulin and glucose levels after a meal affect glucose economy at both hepatic and muscular sites, and plasma insulin concentrations rarely achieve the high and steady levels seen after exogenous insulin infusion in the euglycemic hyperinsulinemic clamp. The minimal model approach was increasingly used in many clinical studies during the last few years but its application to the study of type 2 diabetes remains scarce up to now [21, 30].

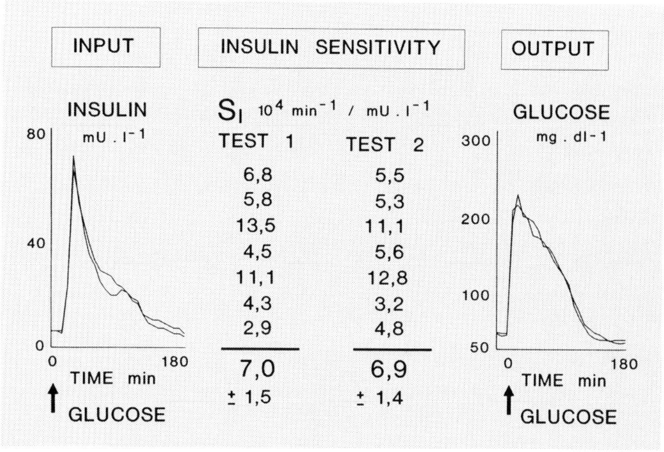

Fig. 2. Illustration of the principle of the frequently sampled intravenous glucose tolerance test (FSIVGTT) analyzed with the minimal model method. Seven healthy young male lean volunteers were submitted to two FSIVGTTs (0.3 g glucose/kg), 1 week apart, in order to study the reproducibility of the index of insulin sensitivity (S_i).

Application to the Study of Type 2 Diabetes

The most conclusive documentation of insulin resistance in obesity and type 2 diabetes has come from studies that have employed the euglycemic hyperinsulinemic glucose clamp technique [reviewed in 6, 8, 9, 26, 36, 37].

We measured the glucose disposal and the endogenous glucose production during euglycemic glucose clamps performed at various plasma insulin levels in order to compare the characteristics of the dose-response curves in nondiabetic obese subjects and in type 2 diabetic patients with those obtained in lean healthy volunteers (fig. 3) [38–42]. The insulin-mediated glucose disposal curve was slightly but significantly shifted to the right in the nondiabetic obese subjects; however, in the diabetic patients, the right shift was more obvious and the highest response was markedly reduced even when supraphysiological plasma insulin levels (above 700 $mU \cdot l^{-1}$) were tested.

Basal hepatic glucose output was similar in lean and obese nondiabetic subjects (around $2\ mg \cdot kg^{-1} \cdot min^{-1}$). However, a complete inhibition by insulin required significantly higher plasma insulin concentrations in obese than in lean subjects. In the type 2 diabetic subjects, hepatic glucose output was significantly increased (above $3\ mg \cdot kg^{-1} \cdot min^{-1}$) after an overnight fast despite simultaneous higher basal plasma insulin levels; moreover, a complete inhibition of the hepatic glucose output was only observed for much higher plasma insulin levels than

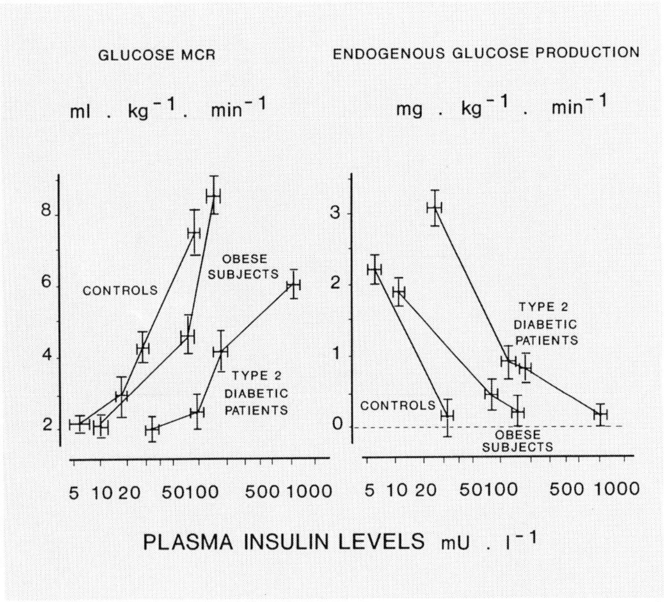

Fig. 3. Dose-response curves of either the MCR of glucose (**a**) or the endogenous glucose production (**b**) versus the plasma insulin levels measured in the basal state and during euglycemic hyperinsulinemic glucose clamps in three groups of subjects: lean controls (n = 8), nondiabetic obese subjects (n = 10) and obese patients with type 2 diabetes mellitus (n = 10).

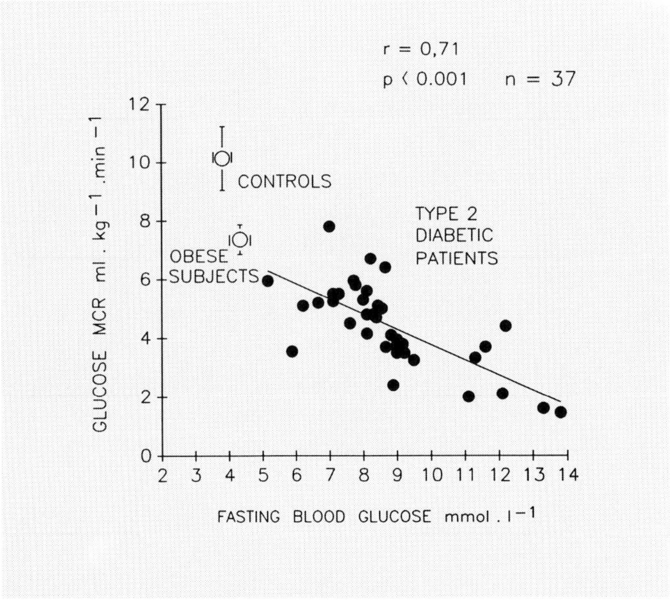

Fig. 4. Relationship between the MCR of glucose measured during a euglycemic hyperinsulinemic glucose clamp (insulin delivery rate: 100 mU·kg^{-1}·h^{-1}) and the fasting blood glucose levels in three groups of subjects: lean controls (mean ± SEM; n = 15), nondiabetic obese subjects (mean ± SEM; n = 16) and type 2 diabetic patients (n = 37).

those necessary in lean and even obese nondiabetic subjects [43, 44].

These results confirm that the obese subjects already have significant insulin resistance at the muscle and hepatic sites but that these abnormalities become much more marked in the diabetic patients [6, 23, 26, 36, 37, 44, 45]. The reduction in insulin sensitivity (increased ED_{50} or reduced K_m), which corresponds to a defect at the receptor level, seems to be predominant in the obese subjects; in contrast, the lower maximal metabolic response (V_{max}), which corresponds to a defect at the postreceptor level, appears to be predominant in the diabetic patients [26].

In order to verify that the peripheral insulin resistance is an early defect in the natural history of type 2 diabetes [9], we measured the glucose MCR during a euglycemic hyperinsulinemic glucose clamp (100 mU·kg^{-1}·h^{-1}) in three groups of subjects: 15 lean controls, 16 nondiabetic obese subjects and 37 patients with mild diabetes whose fasting blood glucose levels under diet therapy alone ranged from 5.2 to 13.8 mmol·l^{-1} (fig. 4). The glucose MCR was significantly lower in the obese than in the lean nondiabetic subjects: 7.5 ± 0.5 vs. 10.2 ± 1.1 ml·kg^{-1}·min^{-1}; $p < 0.05$. The glucose MCR was much more reduced in the type 2 diabetic patients: 4.0 ± 0.3 ml·kg^{-1}·min^{-1}; $p < 0.001$. Moreover, in this population, there was a remarkable inverse relationship between glucose MCR measured during the clamp and fasting blood glucose levels: $r = -0.71$; $p < 0.001$. This indicates that the higher the blood glucose level, the lower the efficacy of insulin to stimulate muscular glucose disposal. The defect in glucose utilization, more particularly the storage to glycogen [46], appears to be an early and important defect in the natural history of type 2 diabetes mellitus [47]. However, the question to know if the muscular defect is predominant on the hepatic defect remains controversial [48].

Finally, we measured the insulin-mediated glucose disposal during a euglycemic hyperinsulinemic clamp (100 mU insulin·kg^{-1}·h^{-1}) in lean healthy volunteers, in obese nondiabetic subjects and in four groups of patients with type 2 diabetes separated by the presence or absence of obesity (BMI > 28 kg/m^2) and by the evolution or not to insulin requirement to achieve acceptable glycemic control (fig. 5) [38–42]. Insulin sensitivity was markedly and significantly reduced in all groups of diabetic subjects when compared with that of lean or obese controls. The

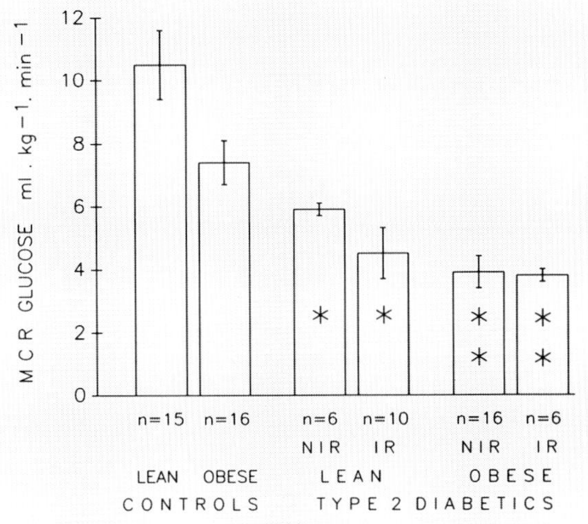

Fig. 5. Comparison of the MCR of glucose measured during a euglycemic hyperinsulinemic glucose clamp (insulin delivery rate: $100\ mU \cdot kg^{-1} \cdot h^{-1}$) in lean and obese subjects (controls), and in four groups of type 2 diabetic patients: noninsulin-requiring (NIR) or insulin-requiring (IR) lean patients, and NIR or IR obese patients. The results are expressed by the mean ± SEM. The asterisks indicate significant differences versus reference values obtained in control subjects: * $p < 0.05$ versus lean controls; ** $p < 0.05$ versus obese controls.

presence of obesity slightly but significantly reduced the insulin-mediated glucose disposal and thus further aggravated insulin resistance [49]. However, the transition to insulin requirement was in most cases not explained by a further decrease in insulin sensitivity but rather by a profound exhaustion of endogenous insulin secretion [50].

When patients with type 2 diabetes first present to a physician, most have had weight excess for several decades and diabetes already for many years, and defects in both insulin action and insulin secretion are present [6, 9, 37, 51, 52]. At this stage, it is impossible to define which defect came first in the evolution of their disease. However, it seems likely that in any given diabetic patient, whatever defect initiates the disturbance in glucose metabolism, it will eventually be followed by the emergence of its counterpart. A lot of evidence demonstrates that receptor/postreceptor insulin defect and B-cell exhaustion can aggravate insulin deficiency and insulin resistance, respectively, through the common step of prolonged hyperglycemia, whether induced by one or the other primary defect [reviewed in 53]. This new concept is known as glucotoxicity [reviewed in 54]. Once it develops, either from insulin deficiency or from insulin resistance, hyperglycemia will exacerbate both defects, thereby closing a pathologic feedback loop [9, 53, 54].

Conclusions

The evidence is overwhelming that diminished insulin sensitivity, i.e. insulin resistance, is present in many pathophysiological states and is thus an important metabolic parameter to be measured [2, 4, 5]. Numerous methods have been proposed over the last five decades to assess insulin sensitivity in vivo and the most important ones have been briefly described in the present review. Each method has its advantages and its disadvantages. For large clinical application, the measure of insulin sensitivity should be obtainable with a reasonable effort, in a limited time period, with minimal risk to the subject. Furthermore, the measure should be sufficiently accurate and precise as to allow intra-subject (to test the effect of a treatment for instance) and inter-subject (to compare various populations) comparison [14]. However, other criteria should also be met to have a gold standard measure. The ideal method should require little specialized equipment and no highly skilled staff; moreover, the attainment of a steady state before a measurement can be made should not be essential, the measure should be independent of the plasma levels of glucose and insulin and reflect sensitivity in the physiological range of insulin action, and, last but not least, the method should be free from any bias that the investigator could introduce [28]. Finally, and ideally, the measure should not be confounded by, but should provide an assessment of, insulin-independent glucose disappearance and should also provide insight into the cellular mechanisms responsible for alterations in insulin sensitivity [14, 36, 55]. As emphasized by Bergman et al. [14], none of the available methods satisfy all criteria, and it is likely that no single measure will ever do.

The most commonly used technique, and now considered as the reference method, is the euglycemic hyperinsulinemic clamp. It has been extensively used in type 2 diabetic patients and has provided huge amounts of interesting data. This is particularly the case when it is performed at various insulin levels in order to study the whole dose-response curve, and when it is coupled with isotopic determination of glucose fluxes and with indirect calorimetry for studying the metabolic fate of glucose. The application of these techniques in the study of patients with type 2 diabetes has clearly demonstrated that insulin resistance plays a major role, both at the liver and the muscles sites, and that the defect in insulin action predominates at the postreceptor level [6, 8, 9, 26, 36, 37]. Nevertheless, the important question of which is the primary defect in type 2 diabetes, the defect in insulin action or that in insulin secretion, still remains a matter of active research and spirited controversy [47, 53, 56, 57].

Acknowledgments

We are indebted to Drs M. Castillo (Granada, Spain), G. Paolisso (Naples, Italy) and B. Jandrain (Liège, Belgium) for their help during the various experimental protocols with the glucose clamp technique. We thank Ms M. Jehasse for secretarial support.

References

1 Turner RC, Rudenski AS, Holman RR, Matthews DR, O'Rahilly SP: Quantitative modelling of endocrine diseases as exemplified by diabetes. Clin Endocrinol (Oxf) 1987;26:107–116.

2 Moller DE, Flier JS: Insulin resistance. Mechanisms, syndromes, and implications. N Engl J Med 1991;325:938–948.

3 Ader M, Bergman RN: Insulin sensitivity in the intact organism. Baillieres Clin Endocrinol Metab 1987;1:879–910.

4 Reaven GM: Role of insulin resistance in human disease. Diabetes 1988;37:1595–1607.

5 DeFronzo RA, Ferrannini E: Insulin resistance: A multifaceted syndrome responsible for NIDDM, obesity, hypertension, dyslipidemia, and atherosclerotic cardiovascular disease. Diabetes Care 1991;14:173–194.

6 DeFronzo RA, Ferrannini E, Koivisto V: New concepts in the pathogenesis and treatment of noninsulin-dependent diabetes mellitus. Am J Med 1983;75:52–81.

7 Reaven GM: Insulin-resistance in noninsulin-dependent diabetes mellitus: Does it exist and can it be measured? Am J Med 1983;74(suppl): 3–17.

8 Gerich JE: Role of insulin resistance in the pathogenesis of type 2 (non-insulin-dependent) diabetes mellitus. Baillieres Clin Endocrinol Metab 1988;2:307–326.

9 DeFronzo RA: The triumvirate: B-cell, muscle, liver. A collusion responsible for NIDDM. Diabetes 1988;37:667–687.

10 Garvey WT: Insulin resistance and noninsulin-dependent diabetes mellitus: Which horse is pulling the cart? Diabetes Metab Rev 1989;5: 727–742.

11 Himsworth HP: Diabetes mellitus. Its differentiation into insulin-sensitive and insulin-insensitive types. Lancet 1936;i:127–130.

12 Yalow RS, Berson SA: Plasma insulin concentrations in nondiabetic and early diabetic subjects. Determination by a new sensitive immunoassay technique. Diabetes 1960;9:254–260.

13 Karam JH, Grodsky GM, Forsham PH: Excessive insulin response to glucose in obese subjects as measured by immunochemical assay. Diabetes 1963;12:197–204.

14 Bergman RN, Finegood DT, Ader M: Assessment of insulin sensitivity in vivo. Endocr Rev 1985;6:45–86.

15 Shen SW, Reaven GM, Farquhar JW: Comparison of impedance to insulin-mediated glucose uptake in normal subjects and in subjects with latent diabetes. J Clin Invest 1970;49:2151–2160.

16 Andres R, Swerdloff R, Pozefsky T, Coleman D: Manual feedback technique for the control of blood glucose concentration; in Skeggs LT Jr (ed): Automation in Analytical Chemistry. New York Mediad Inc, 1966, pp 486–491.

17 DeFronzo RA, Tobin JD, Andres R: Glucose clamp technique: A method for quantifying insulin secretion and resistance. Am J Physiol 1979;232:E214–E223.

18 Steele R: Influences of glucose loading and of injected insulin on hepatic glucose output. Ann NY Acad Sci 1959;82:420–430.

19 Wolfe RR (ed): Tracers in Metabolic Research. Radioisotope and Stable Isotope/Mass Spectrometry Methods. New York, Liss, 1984.

20 Alberti KGMM, Home PD, Taylor R (eds): Techniques for metabolic investigation in man. Baillieres Clin Endocrinol Metab 1987;1: 773–1076.

21 Bergman RN, Hope ID, Yang YJ, Watanabe RM, Meador MA, Youn JH, Ader M: Assessment of insulin sensitivity in vivo: A critical review. Diabetes Metab Rev 1989;5:411–429.

22 Felber JP, Golay A, Felley C, Jequier E: Regulation of glucose storage in obesity and diabetes: Metabolic aspects. Diabetes Metab Rev 1988;4:691–700.

23 Groop LC, Bonadonna RC, DelPrato S, Ratheiser K, Zyck K, Ferrannini E, DeFronzo RA: Glucose and free fatty acid metabolism in non-insulin-dependent diabetes mellitus. Evidence for multiple sites of insulin resistance. J Clin Invest 1989;84:205–213.

24 Ferrannini E: The theoretical bases of indirect calorimetry: A review. Metabolism 1988;37: 287–301.

25 Kahn CR: Insulin resistance, insulin sensitivity, and insulin unresponsiveness: A necessary distinction. Metabolism 1978;27:1893–1902.

26 Kolterman OG, Gray RS, Griffin J, Burstein P, Insel J, Scarlett JA, Olefsky JM: Receptor and postreceptor defects contribute to the insulin resistance in noninsulin-dependent diabetes mellitus. J Clin Invest 1981;68:957–969.

27 Scheen AJ, Castillo M, Paolisso G, Jandrain B, Lefèbvre PJ: Normal feedback inhibition of insulin secretion by insulin but reduced metabolic clearance rate of the hormone in obese subjects; in Ailhaud G, Guy-Grand B, Lafontan M, Ricquier D (eds): Obesity in Europe 91. London, Libbey, 1992, pp 201–205.

28 Ng LL: Application of modelling techniques to the assessment of insulin sensitivity in man. Diabetic Med 1988;5:217–222.

29 Cobelli C, Bergman RN (eds): Carbohydrate Metabolism. Quantitative Physiology and Mathematical Modelling. Chichester, Wiley, 1981.

30 Bergman RN: Toward physiological understanding of glucose tolerance. Minimal-model approach. Diabetes 1989;38:1512–1527.

31 Rudenski AS, Matthews DR, Levy JC, Turner RC: Understanding 'insulin resistance': Both glucose resistance and insulin resistance are required to model human diabetes. Metabolism 1991;40:908–917.

32 Matthews DR, Hosker JP, Rudenski AS, Naylor BA, Treacher DF, Turner RC: Homeostasis model assessment: Insulin resistance and B-cell function from fasting plasma glucose and insulin concentrations in man. Diabetologia 1985; 28:412–419.

33 Hosker JP, Matthews DR, Rudenski AS, Burnett MA, Darling P, Bown EG, Turner RC: Continuous infusion of glucose with model assessment: Measurement of insulin resistance and B-cell function in man. Diabetologia 1985; 28:401–411.

34 Bergman RN, Phillips LS, Cobelli C: Physiologic evaluation of factors controlling glucose tolerance in man. Measurement of insulin sensitivity and B-cell glucose sensitivity from the response to intravenous glucose. J Clin Invest 1981;68:1456–1467.

35 Caumo A, Giacca A, Morgese M, Pozza G, Micossi P, Cobelli C: Minimal models of glucose disappearance: Lessons from the labelled IVGTT. Diabetic Med 1991;8:822–832.

36 Garvey WT, Kolterman OG: Correlation of in vivo and in vitro actions of insulin in obesity and noninsulin-dependent diabetes mellitus: Role of the glucose transport system. Diabetes Metab Rev 1988;4:543–569.

37 Lillioja S, Bogardus C: Obesity and insulin resistance: Lessons learned from the Pima Indians. Diabetes Metab Rev 1988;4:517–540.
38 Castillo M, Scheen AJ, Lefèbvre P, Luyckx A: Insulin-stimulated glucose disposal is not increased in anorexia nervosa. J Clin Endocrinol Metab 1985;60:311–314.
39 Jandrain B, Scheen AJ, Henrivaux P, Paolisso G, Luyckx AS, Lefèbvre PJ: Insulin sensitivity and glucose tolerance during the menstrual cycle; in Vague J, Björntorp P, Guy-Grand B, Rebuffé-Scrive M, Vague P (eds): Metabolic Complications of Human Obesities. Amsterdam, Excerpta Medica, 1985, ICS No 682, pp 241–247.
40 Paolisso G, Sgambato S, Giugliano D, Torella R, Varricchio M, Scheen AJ, D'Onofrio F, Lefèbvre PJ: Impaired insulin-induced erythrocyte magnesium accumulation is correlated to impaired insulin-mediated glucose disposal in type 2 (non-insulin-dependent) diabetic patients. Diabetologia 1988;31:910–915.
41 Scheen AJ, Castillo M, Lefèbvre PJ: Insulin sensitivity in anorexia nervosa – A mirror image of obesity? Diabetes Metab Rev 1988;4: 681–690.
42 Scheen AJ, Paolisso G, Salvatore T, Lefèbvre PJ: Improvement of insulin-induced glucose disposal in obese patients with NIDDM after 1-week treatment with *d*-fenfluramine. Diabetes Care 1991;14:325–332.
43 DeFronzo RA, Ferrannini E: Regulation of hepatic glucose metabolism in humans. Diabetes Metab Rev 1987;3:415–459.
44 Ferrannini E, Groop LC: Hepatic glucose production in insulin-resistant states. Diabetes Metab Rev 1989;5:711–725.
45 DeFronzo RA, Gunnarsson R, Bjorkman O, Olsson M, Wahren J: Effects of insulin on peripheral and splanchnic glucose metabolism in noninsulin-dependent (type II) diabetes mellitus. J Clin Invest 1985;76:149–155.
46 Shulman GI, Rothman DL, Jue T, Stein P, DeFronzo RA, Shulman RG: Quantitation of muscle glycogen synthesis in normal subjects and subjects with non-insulin-dependent diabetes by ^{13}C-nuclear magnetic resonance spectroscopy. N Engl J Med 1990;322:223–228.
47 DeFronzo RA: Pathogenesis of type 2 (non-insulin-dependent) diabetes mellitus: A balanced overview. Diabetologia 1992;35:389–397.
48 Gerich JE: Is muscle the major site of insulin resistance in type 2 (non-insulin-dependent) diabetes mellitus? Diabetologia 1991;34:607–610.
49 Scheen AJ, Paolisso G, Castillo M, Jandrain B, Lefèbvre PJ: Modest but significant influence of obesity in the reduction of insulin-induced glucose disposal in type 2 diabetes melitus. Int J Obes 1991;15(suppl 1):42.
50 Groop L, Schalin C, Franssila-Kallunki A, Widen E, Ekstrand A, Eriksson J: Characteristics of non-insulin-dependent diabetic patients with secondary failure to oral antidiabetic therapy. Am J Med 1989;87:183–190.
51 Scheen A, Nemery A, Luyckx A, Lefèbvre P: Etiologie et physiopathologie des diabètes sucrés. Encycl Méd Chir (Paris, France), Glandes-Nutrition, 10366 C^{10}, 2-1986, 18 p.
52 Scheen AJ: From obesity to type 2 diabetes. Acta Clin Belg 1992;47(suppl 14):30–36.
53 Scheen AJ, Paquot N, Lefèbvre PJ: La cellule B dans le diabète de type II: Coupable ou victime? In Journées Annuelles de Diabétologie de l'Hôtel-Dieu. Paris, Flammarion Médecine-Sciences, 1991, pp 153–169.
54 Rossetti L, Giaccari A, DeFronzo RA: Glucose toxicity. Diabetes Care 1990;13:610–630.
55 Olefsky JM, Garvey WT, Henry RR, Brillon D, Matthaei S, Freidenberg GR: Cellular mechanisms of insulin resistance in non-insulin-dependent (type II) diabetes. Am J Med 1988; 85(suppl 5A):86–105.
56 Turner RC, Matthews DR, Clark A, O'Rahilly S, Rudenski AS, Levy J: Pathogenesis of NIDDM – A disease of deficient insulin secretion. Baillieres Clin Endocrinol Metab 1988;2: 327–342.
57 Mitrakou A, Kelley D; Mokan M, Veneman T, Pangburn T, Reilly J, Gerich J: Role of reduced suppression of glucose production and diminished early insulin release in impaired glucose tolerance. N Engl J Med 1992;326:22–29.

Horm Res 1992;38:28–32

P. Vague
D. Raccah

Service d'Endocrinologie, Métabolisme et Nutrition, CHU La Timone, Marseille, France

The Syndrome of Insulin Resistance

Key Words
Insulin resistance
Cardiovascular disease
Obesity

Abstract
It is well known that excessive weight is associated with resistance to insulin-mediated glucose uptake and predisposition to the development of type II diabetes. It has been shown more recently that excessive weight and insulin resistance tend to be associated to android fat distribution, arterial hypertension, elevated levels of triglycerides, low concentration of HDL cholesterol and defective fibrinolysis. The terms syndrome of insulin resistance, metabolic syndrome or syndrome X have been proposed to describe this cluster of abnormalities. The pathophysiological mechanisms which could explain the interrelations between these different parameters are still only partly understood. Epidemiological prospective studies have demonstrated that the metabolic syndrome is a risk factor for coronary heart disease and type II diabetes. The mechanisms involved in the development of diabetes are relatively well established, but those which are implicated in the atherothrombotic process are far from being cleary described. Anyway, sufficient presumption exists to attempt at decreasing insulin resistance when it exists. Physical training and, if indicated, weight reduction are the simplest means.

Insulin resistance may be secondary to various diseases such as Cushing's disease and acromegaly. In these conditions well-known mechanisms counteract the action of insulin. Primary and well-characterized states of insulin resistance also exist with an abnormal interaction between insulin and its receptor.

In addition to these relatively rare and exceptional conditions, resistance to insulin-mediated glucose disposal is a frequent finding in the general population and is more or less related to an excess of body weight. Its mechanism is not entirely understood. However, two different approaches have shown that insulin resistance may be responsible for a 'metabolic syndrome' and may have deleterious implications especially in predisposing to noninsulin-dependent diabetes mellitus (NIDDM) and cardiovascular disease (CVD). The first approach based on anthropometry and epidemiology has shown that obesity (of a particular body fat distribution) associated with a high level of plasma insulin is a risk factor for NIDDM and CVD [1–3]. The second has focused on the relationship between resistance to insulin-mediated glucose uptake and NIDDM, CVD, and arterial hypertension [4].

In this brief review, we will first discuss and describe the insulin resistance syndrome. The relationships be-

Prof. Ph. Vague
Service de Médecine Interne et Nutrition
CHU La Timone
bd Jean-Moulin
F–13385 Marseille Cedex 5 (France)

tween the various observed abnormalities will then be analyzed. Finally, the responsibility of this syndrome in the predisposition to diabetes and CVD will be discussed.

The Insulin Resistance Syndrome: Does It Exist?

The resistance to insulin-mediated glucose uptake may be estimated in man by both simple and complex techniques [5]. In the presence of normal blood glucose values, resistance to insulin action must be accompanied by a proportional compensatory increase in plasma insulin concentration. In other words, among nondiabetic subjects insulin resistance is associated with a proportional hyperinsulinemia [6]. Therefore, in studies dealing with a limited number of individuals, resistance to insulin action may be directly estimated. In larger studies, however, the measurements of plasma insulin either fasting of after a standard glucose load are easier to determine and are used to estimate insulin resistance indirectly.

Given this background, it has been demonstrated directly and indirectly by measuring plasma insulin that insulin resistance is associated with various clinical, metabolic and hormonal characteristics. At the clinical level, a direct relationship exists between the relative weight and the resistance to insulin action. This phenomenon has been known for a long time and was first described when insulin assay became available [7, 8]. However, for a given relative weight individual differences in insulin sensitivity are important. The distribution of body fat varies according to sex in adult individuals. In men, fat tissue is proportionally less abundant than in women [9, 10], it predominates in the upper part of the body [9, 11] and in splanchnic tissues [11, 12]. Various anthropometric techniques have been used to estimate the localization of body fat. The simplest and probably the most discriminant is the determination of the ratio between the waist and the hip girths [13]. The higher the ratio, the more abundant is the proportion of visceral fat, and the lower the proportion of subcutaneous fat. It has been shown that for a given relative body weight insulin resistance and plasma insulin concentration are positively correlated with the waist-to-hip girth ratio, at least in women [14].

Individuals with essential hypertension are insulin-resistant [15–20], and this resistance is proportional to the systolic and diastolic pressure level [18].

Abnormalities in the disposal of metabolic substrates are associated with insulin resistance, mainly glucose intolerance [21] and elevated concentrations of VLDL triglycerides [22]. However, more subtle anormalities such as high concentration of LDL cholesterol and apoprotein B, and low concentrations of HDL cholesterol, HDL_2 cholesterol and apoprotein A_1, are part of an atherogenic lipidic profile described in association with upper body fat distribution [23–26].

In women a hyperandrogenic state characterized by a low level of sex hormone-binding globulin, high concentration of free testosterone and sometimes polycystic ovary syndrome is associated with android fat distribution, insulin resistance and hyperinsulinemia [27–30].

Finally, defective fibrinolysis was first described more than 20 years ago in obese subjects [31, 32]. Recently it has been demonstrated that in various groups including normal subjects [33], obese subjects [34], NIDDM patients [35] and patients with angina pectoris [36] a positive relationship exists between plasma insulin and plasminogen activator inhibitor-1 (PAI-1), the major inhibitor and regulator of the fibrinolytic system in vivo [37]. PAI-1 probably plays an important role in the development of the atherothrombotic process [38, 39] and has been described as an independent risk marker for CVD [40–45].

All of the various abnormalities cited above seem to cluster in the same individual [9, 46]. This clinical impression is confirmed by two studies. The first, dealing with a sample of around 500 nondiabetic, 40- to 50-years-old obese patients, demonstrated a positive correlation between the waist-to-hip girth ratio on the one hand and plasma insulin, glucose, triglyceride, uric acid concentration and systolic and diastolic blood pressure on the other [47]. In the second, a population-based study (The San Antonio Heart Study), body fat mass and distribution, glucose tolerance, blood pressure, serum lipids and plasma insulin were all shown to be closely associated [46].

Therefore, it seems justified to describe a syndrome of insulin resistance. Reaven [48] has coined the term 'syndrome X', to describe the aggregation of high blood pressure, glucose intolerance, hyperinsulinemia and an unfavorable lipid profile. A strong argument could be put forward to add upper body fat distribution and defective fibrinolysis to this syndrome of insulin resistance [49].

Relationship between the Facets of the Insulin Resistance Syndrome

In this constellation, clinical, hormonal and metabolic abnormalities are interrelated according to various mechanisms, the majority of which to date not been entirely elucidated. Some may merely represent an association but some abnormalities may be primary and others the consequence of these.

A genetic predisposition appeared to be not only involved in the control of body weight, but also in the amount of body fat and its distribution [50], in insulin resistance [51, 52], in the susceptibility to hypertension [53] and hypertriglyceridemia [54]. From a theoretical point of view the clustering of these abnormalities could simply be secondary to a common genetic predisposition in relation to a linkage disequilibrium.

However, although insulin resistance could be partly genetic in origin [51, 52] it is mainly secondary to the excessive body weight as it evolves in parallel with weight change [55, 56]. Fat mass distribution has a strong genetic determination [50]. It has been postulated that visceral fat accumulation could induce an insulin-resistance state [57]. Less sensitive to the lipolytic action of insulin, visceral fat tissue delivers a large flux of free fatty acids in the portal circulation. This flux may increase hepatic neoglycogenesis and lipoprotein synthesis, diminish hepatic insulin clearance and through the Randle's circle induce resistance to insulin-mediated glucose uptake in liver and muscle tissue.

Hyperglyceridemia is mainly the consequence of an exaggerated hepatic synthesis of triglyceride under the influence of both high insulin impregnation and concomitant presence of glucose and free fatty acid fluxes [58]. The low concentration of HDL cholesterol is directly due to the excess of VLDL triglyceride occurring by well-known mechanisms.

The elevated PAI-1 levels and as a consequence the fibrinolytic defect appear secondary to the resistance to insulin action and the compensatory hyperinsulinism. In fact, attempts to decrease insulin resistance (increasing insulin sensitivity) by moderate weight loss [59–62], physical excercise [63, 64] and metformin treatment [65] are accompanied by an improvement in blood PAI-1 levels. However, the mechanisms linking hyperinsulinemia and increased PAI synthesis is still unclear [for review, see 66].

It has been suggested mainly on experimental grounds that high blood pressure could be a consequence of insulin resistance. Fructose-fed rats develop insulin resistance and hypertension. In physically trained rats insulin resistance does not appear and hypertension does not develop [67]. The compensatory hyperinsulinemia could result in an exaggerated sodium tubular reabsorption and an increase in adrenergic tone [18]. However, patients presenting with insulinoma are not hypertensive [68].

At the present time, while it has been well demonstrated that all the above described abnormalities tend to cluster together, and that a syndrome (association of symptoms and/or signs) can be described, it is fair to state that in terms of pathophysiological interrelations, the global picture is far from complete.

Possible Consequences of the Syndrome of Insulin Resistance

It has been known for sometime that obesity, especially with android distribution, could be a risk factor for type 2 diabetes and the clinical manifestation of atherosclerosis [1]. It has been well established from prospective studies that android fat distribution is, at least in men, associated with an increased risk of developing type 2 diabetes [3]. Populations with a high prevalence of diabetes such as Micronesians, Pima Indians or Hispano-Americans are characterized by a fairly high prevalence of obesity and hyperinsulinemia [69]. Among Nauruans, those who develop diabetes are those who present with hyperinsulinemia [70]. Although the genetic abnormalities making an individual susceptible to become diabetic are largely unknown, it is tempting to think that diabetes will supervene in subjects of whom the β cells are unable to cope with an increasing demand of insulin to compensate for insulin resistance.

Three epidemiological prospective studies have shown that a high concentration of plasma insulin is a risk factor for CVD [71–73]. Among type 2 diabetic patients, those presenting with hyperinsulinemia are likely to develop ECG abnormalities within 5 years [74]. These studies lend strong support to Stout's theory suggesting that insulin could be atherogenic. The fact that hyperinsulinemia is the hallmark of the insulin resistance syndrome which includes many well-known risk factors for CVD helps to understand why such an association has been found but does not allow us to conclude that hyperinsulinemia or insulin resistance are directly responsible for the development of the atherogenic process.

A direct role for insulin in the atherogenic process has been severely criticized [75]. The two main reasons are: (1) there is no dose-effect relationship between insulinemia and risk of CHD in the prospective studies, the risk being confined to the subjects in the upper quintile or decile of insulinemia, and (2) so many confounding variables exist that their potential role cannot be eliminated even by sophisticated statistical analysis.

Whatever the mechanisms involved, it can however be clearly stated that subjects with the insulin resistance syndrome do present a constellation of atherogenic abnormalities and that hyperinsulinemia is at least a marker of other risk factors for CVD.

Given that the high prevalence of this syndrome in the population may be higher than that of isolated hypercholesterolemia, it is important in terms of public health to determine by prospective studies whether by decreasing insulin resistance one can prevent CVD. Under such circumstances the role of insulin resistance in the atherosclerotic process would be demonstrated. Such studies are in progress [76].

References

1 Vague J: The degree of masculine differentiation of obesities. A factor determining predisposition to diabetes, atherosclerosis gout and uric calculous disease. Am J Clin Nutr 1956;4: 20–28.
2 Vague P, Boeuf G, Depieds R, Vague J: Plasma insulin levels in human obesity; in Vague J (ed): Physiopathology of Adipose Tissue. Amsterdam, Excerpta Medica Foundation, 1969, pp 203–225.
3 Larsson BO: Obesity and prospective risk for associated diseases; in Vague J, Björntorp P, Guy-Grand B, Rebuffé-Scrive M, Vague P (eds): Metabolic Complications of Human Obesities. Amsterdam, Elsevier, 1989, pp 21–29.
4 Reaven GM: Role of insulin resistance in human disease. Diabetes 1988;37:1595–1607.
5 Del Prato S, Ferrannini E, Defronzo R: Evaluation of insulin sensitivity in men; in Clarks, Larsen, Porte (eds): Methods in Diabetes Research. New York, Wiley, 1986, vol 2, pp 35–76.
6 Olefsky J, Farquhar JW, Reaven G: Relationship between fasting plasma insulin level and resistance to insulin-mediated glucose uptake in normal and diabetic subjects. Diabetes 1973;22:507–513.
7 Yalow RJ, Blick IM, Roth J, Berson SA: Plasma insulin and growth hormone in obesity and diabetes. Ann NY Acad Sci 1965;131:357–373.
8 Bagdade J, Bierman EL, Porte D: The significance of basal insulin levels in the evaluation of the insulin response to glucose in diabetic and non-diabetic subjects. J Clin Invest 1967;19: 475–482.
9 Vague J: Obesities. Marseille, Libbey & Solal, 1991, pp 1–153.
10 Bishop CW: References values for arm muscle area, arm fat area, subscapular skinfold thickness, and sum of skinfold thickness for American adults. J Parenter Enter Nutr 1984;8:515–522.
11 Sjöstrom L, Kvist H, Tylen U: Methodological aspects of measurements of adipose tissue distribution; in Vague J, et al (eds): Metabolic Complications of Human Obesities. Amsterdam, Elsevier, 1989, pp 13–19.
12 Dixon AK: Abdominal fat assessed by computed tomography: Sex difference in distribution. Clin Radiol 1983;34:189–191.
13 Bjorntorp P: The associations between obesity adipose tissue distribution and diseases. Acta Med Scand 1978;723 (suppl):121–134.
14 Vague P, Juhan-Vague I, Chabert V, Alessi MC, Atlan C: Fat distribution and plasminogen activator inhibitor activity is non-diabetic obese women. Metabolism 1989;9:913–915.
15 Welborn TA, Brenckenridge A, Rubinstein AH, Dollery CT, Fraser TR: Serum-insulin in essential hypertension and in peripheral vascular disease. Lancet 1966;i:1336–1337.
16 Modan M, Halkin H, Almog S, Lusky A, Eshkh A Shefi M, Shitrit A, Fuchs A: Hyperinsulinemia: A link between hypertension, obesity and glucose intolerance. J Clin Invest 1985;75:809–817.
17 Manicardi V, Cambellini L, Bellodi G, Coscelli C, Ferrannini E: Evidence for an association of high blood pressure and hyperinsulinemia in obese man. J Clin Endocrinol Metab 1986;62: 1302–1304.
18 Ferrannini E, Buzzigoli G, Bonadonna R, Giorico MA, Oleggini M, Graziadei L, Pedrinelli R, Brandi L, Bevilacqua S: Insulin resistance in essential hypertension. N Engl J Med 1987; 317:350–356.
19 Shen DC, Shieh SM, Fuh M, Wu DA, Chen YDI, Reaven GM: Resistance to insulin-stimulated glucose uptake in patients with hypertension. J Clin Endocrinol Metab 1988;66:580–583.
20 Bonora E, Zavaroni I, Alpi O, Pezzarossa A, Bruschi F, Dall'Aglio E, Guerra L, Coscelli C, Butturini U: Relationship between blood pressure and plasma insulin in non-obese and obese non-diabetic subjects. Diabetologia 1987;30: 719–723.
21 Reaven GM, Hollenbeck CB, Chien YDI: Relationship between glucose tolerance, insulin secretion, and insulin action in non-obese individuals with varying degrees of glucose tolerance. Diabetologia 1989;32:52–55.
22 Reaven GM, Chen YDI: Role of insulin in regulation of lipoprotein metabolism in diabetes. Diabetes Metab Rev 1988;44:639–652.
23 Barakat HA, Burton DS, Carpenter JW, Holden D, Israel RG: Body fat distribution, plasma lipoproteins and the risks of coronary heart disease of male subjects. Int J Obes 1988; 12:473–480.
24 Desires JP, Mourjani S, Ferland M, Tremblay A, Lupien JP, Nadeau A, et al: Adipose tissue distribution and plasma lipoprotein levels in obese women. Importance of intra-abdominal fat. Atherosclerosis 1989;9:203–210.
25 Peeples LM, Carpenter JW, Israel RG, Barakat MA: Alterations in low density lipoproteins in subjects with abdominal obesity. Metabolism 1989;35:1029–1036.
26 Ostlund RE, Staten M, Kormt WM, Schultz J, Malley M: The ratio of waist-to-hip circumference, plasma insulin level and glucose intolerance as independent predictors of the HDL cholesterol level in older men. Engl J Med 1990;322:229–234.
27 Pugeat M, Crave JC, Elmidani M: Pathophysiology of sex hormone binding globulin: Relation to insulin. J Steroid Biochem Mol Biol 1991;40:841–849.
28 Chang RJ, Nakamura RM, Judd HL, Kaplan SA: Insulin resistance in non-obese patients with polycystic ovarian disease. J Clin Endocrinol Metab 1983;57:356.
29 Shoupe D, Kumar D, Lobo RA: Insulin resistance in polycystic ovary syndrome. Am J Obstet Gynecol 1983;147:588.
30 Burghen GA, Givens JR, Kitabchi AE: Correlation of hyperandrogenism with hyperinsulinism in polycystic ovarian disease. J Clin Endocrinol Metab 1980;50:113–120.
31 Shaw DA, McNaughton D: Relationship between blood fibrinolytic activity and body fatness. Lancet 1963;i:352–354.
32 Ogston DM, Andrew GM: Fibrinolysis in obesity. Lancet 1964;ii:1205–1207.
33 Vague P, Juhan-Vague I, Aillaud MF, Badier C, Viard R, Alessi MC, Collen D: Correlation between blood fribrinolytic activity, plasminogen activator inhibitor level, plasma insulin level and relative body weight in normal and obese subjects. Metabolism 1986;35:250–253.
34 Vague P, Juhan-Vague I, Chabert V, Alessi MC, Atlan C: Fat distribution and plasminogen activator inhibitor activity in non-diabetic obese women. Metabolism 1989;38:913–915.
35 Juhan-Vague I, Roul C, Alessi MC, Ardissone JP, Heim M, Vague P: Increased plasminogen activator inhibitor activity in non-insulin-dependent diabetic patients. Relationship with plasma insulin. Thromb Haemost 1989;61: 370–373.

36 Juhan-Vague I, Alessi MC, Joly P, Thirion X, Vague P, Declerck PJ, Serradimigni A, Collen D: Plasma plasminogen activator inhibitor in angina pectoris. Influence of plasma insulin and acute-phase response. Arteriosclerosis 1989;9:362–367.
37 Bachmann F: Fibrinolysis; in Verstraete M, Vermylen J, Lunen HR, Arnout J (eds): Thrombosis and haemostasis. Leuven, Leuven University Press, 1987, pp 227–265.
38 Niewiarowsky S, Rao K: Contribution of thrombogenic factors to the pathogenesis of atherosclerosis. Prog Cardiovasc Dis 1983;26: 197–222.
39 Schwartz CJ, Valente AJ, Kelly JL, Srague EA, Edwards EH: Thrombosis and development of atherosclerosis: Rokitansky revisited. Thromb Haemost 1988;14:189–195.
40 Davies MJ, Thomas A: Thrombosis and acute coronary artery lesions in sudden cardiac ischemic death. N Engl J Med 1984;310:1137–1140.
41 Paramo JA, Colucci M, Collen D, Van de Werf F: Plasminogen activator inhibitor in the blood of patients with coronary artery disease. Br Med J 1985;291:575–576.
42 Hamsten A, Wiman B, Defaire U, Blomback M: Increased plasma level of a rapid inhibitor of tissue plasminogen activator in young survivors of myocardial infarction. N Engl J Med 1985;313:1557–1563.
43 Meade TW, Broozovic M, Chakrabarti RR, Haines AR, Imeson JD, Mellows S, Miller GJ, North WRS, Stirling J, Thompson SG: Haemostatic function and ischaemic heart disease: Principal results of the Northwick Park Heart Study. Lancet 1986;ii:533–537.
44 Hamsten A, Defaire U, Walldius G, Dahlen G, Szamosi A, Landov C, Blomback M, Wiman B: Plasminogen activator inhibitor in plasma: Risk factor for recurrent myocardial infarction. Lancet 1987;ii:3–9.
45 Metha J, Mahta P, Lawson D, Saldeen T: Plasma tissue plasminogen activator inhibitor levels in coronary artery disease: Correlation with age and serum triglyceride concentrations. J Am Coll Cardiol 1987;9:263–268.
46 Ferrannini E, Haffner SM, Mitchell BD, Stern MP: Hyperinsulinaemia: The key feature of a cardiovascular and metabolic syndrome. Diabetologia 1991;34:416–422.
47 Vague J: Diabetogenic and atherogenic fat; in Domura Y (ed): Progress in Obesity Research. London, Libbey, 1990, vol 1, pp 343–358.
48 Reaven GM: Role of insulin resistance in human disease. Diabetes 1988;37:1495–1607.
49 Vague P: Insulin resistance, a unifying concept. Diabete Metab 1991;17:75–77.
50 Bouchard C: Génétique et obésité chez l'homme. Diabete Metab 1988;14:407–413.
51 Haffner SM, Stern MP, Hazvda H, Mitchell BD, Patterson JN: Increased insulin concentrations in non-diabetic offsprings of diabetic parents. N Engl J Med 1988;219:1297–1301.
52 Laws A, Stefanick M, Reaven G: Insulin resistance and hypertriglyceridemia in non-diabetic relatives of patients with non-insulin-dependent diabetes mellitus. J Clin Endocrinol Metab 1989;69:343–347.
53 Bulpit CJ: Handbock of Hypertension. Amsterdam, Elsevier, 1985.
54 Schaefer EJ, Levy RI: Pathogenesis and management of lipoprotein disorders. N Engl J Med 1985;312:1300–1310.
55 Olefsky JM, Reaven GM, Farquhar JW: Effects of weight reduction on obesity: Studies of carbohydrate and lipid metabolism in normal and hyperlipoproteinemic subjects. J Clin Invest 1974;53:64–76.
56 Golay A, Felber JP, Dusmet M, Gomez F, Curchod B, Jequier E: Effect of weight loss on glucose disposal in obese and obese diabetic patients. Int J Obes 1985;9:181–190.
57 Björntorp P: Metabolic implication of body fat distribution. Diabetes Care 1991;14:1132–1143.
58 Tobey TA, Greenfield M, Kraemer F, Reaven GM: Relationship between insulin resistance, insulin secretion, very low sensitivity lipoprotein kinetics and plasma triglyceride levels in normotriglyceridemic man. Metabolism 1991; 30:165–171.
59 Juhan-Vague I, Alessi MC, Fossat C, Valadier J, Aillaud MF, Serradimigni A: Clinical relevance of high PAI-1 level in patients with idiopathic/recurrent deep venous thrombosis. Fibrinolysis 1988;2(suppl 2):85–88.
60 Sundell IB, Dahlgren S, Ranby M, Lundin E, Stenling R, Nilsson TK: Reduction of elevated plasminogen activator inhibitor levels during modest weight loss. Fibrinolysis 1989;3:51–53.
61 Meharabian M, Peter JB, Barnard RJ, Lusis AJ: Dietary regulation of fibrinolytic factors. Atherosclerosis 1990;84:25–32.
62 Huisweld IA, Leenen R, van den Koopy K, Hospers JEH, Seidell JC, Deurenberg P, Kopeschaar HPF, Mosterd WL, Boupma BN: Body Composition and weight reduction in relation to antigen and activity of plasminogen activator inhibitor (PAI-1) in overweight individuals. Fibrinolysis 1990;4:84–85.
63 Estelles A, Aznar J, Tormo G, Sapena P, Tormo V, Espana F: Influence of a rehabilitation sports program on the fibrinolytic activity of patients after myocardial infarction. Thromb Res 1989;55:203–212.
64 Gris JC, Schved JF, Aguilar-Martinez P, Arnaud A, Sanchez N: Impact of physical training on plasminogen activator inhibitor activity in sedentary men. Fibrinolysis 1990;4:97–98.
65 Vague P, Juhan-Vague I, Alessi MC, Badier C, Valadier J: Metformin decreases the high plasminogen activator inhibitor capacity, plasma insulin and triglyceride levels in non-diabetic obese subjects. Thromb Haemost 1987;57: 326–328.
66 Juhan-Vague I, Alessi MC, Vague P: Increased plasma plasminogen activator inhibitor 1 levels. A possible link between insulin resistance and atherothrombosis. Diabetologia 1991;34: 457–462.
67 Reaven GM: Resistance to insulin-stimulated glucose uptake and hyperinsulinemia. Role in non-insulin-dependent diabetes, high blood pressure, dyslipidemia and coronary heart disease. Diabete Metab 1991;17:78–86.
68 Pontiroli AE, Alberetto M, Pozza G: Patients with insulinoma show insulin resistance in the absence of arterial hypertension. Diabetologia 1992;35:284–285.
69 Haffner SM: Hyperinsulinemia as a possible etiology for the high prevalence of non-insulin-dependent diabetes in Mexican Americans. Diabete Metab 1987;13:337–344.
70 Zimmet P: Non-insulin-dependent diabetes mellitus: Does it really exist? Diabetic Med 1989;6:728–735.
71 Pyorala K: Relationship of glucose tolerance and plasma insulin to the incidence of coronary heart disease. Results from two populations studies in Finland. Diabetes Care 1979;2:131–141.
72 Welborn TA, Weame K: Coronary heart disease incidence and cardiovascular mortality in Busselton with reference to glucose and insulin concentrations. Diabetes Care 1979;2:154–160.
73 Ducimetiere P, Eschwege E, Papoz L, Richard JL, Claude JR, Rosselin G: Relationship of plasma insulin levels to the incidence of myocardial infarction and coronary heart disease mortality in a middle-aged population. Diabetologia 1980;19:205–210.
74 Hockaday TDR, Phil D: Serum insulin concentration and anticipatory factors of cardiomyopathy in NIDDM. Diabete Metab 1987;13:92–98.
75 Jarrett RJ: Is insulin atherogenic? Diabetologia 1988;31:71–75.
76 Fontbonne A, Andre P, Eschwede E, and the Bigpro Study Group: Bigpro (biguanides and the prevention of the risk of obesity) study design. A randomized trial of metformin versus placebo in the correction of the metabolic abnormalities associated with insulin resistance. Diabete Metab 1991;17:249–254.

Horm Res 1992;38:33–38

Philippe Passa

Department of Endocrinology and Diabetology, Hospital Saint-Louis, Paris, France

Hyperinsulinemia, Insulin Resistance and Essential Hypertension

Key Words
Insulinemia
Insulin resistance
Hypertension
Antihypertensive treatment

Abstract

Glucose intolerance and noninsulin-dependent diabetes are commonly associated with hypertension. Epidemiological data suggest that this association is independent of age and obesity. Much evidence indicates that the link between diabetes and essential hypertension is hyperinsulinemia. When hypertensive patients whether obese or of normal weight are compared with matched normotensive control subjects, an increased plasma insulin response to a glucose challenge is consistently observed. Studies using insulin glucose clamp techniques in combination with tracer glucose infusion and indirect calorimetry have demonstrated that the insulin resistance in hypertensive subjects is located in muscles and restricted to glycogen synthesis. The relations between hyperinsulinemia and blood pressure do not prove that the relationship is a causal one. However, at least four mechanisms may link hyperinsulinemia with hypertension: Na^+ retention, sympathetic nervous system overactivity, disturbed membrane ion transport and proliferation of vascular smooth muscle cells. Diuretics and β-blockers may enhance insulin resistance, which is not affected by calcium antagonists, but decreased by the ACE inhibitor captopril. Weight reduction and regular physical exercise can improve insulin sensitivity and decrease blood pressure values. These nonpharmacological interventions should be more strongly recommended to diabetic and nondiabetic hypertensive patients.

Introduction

A few years ago, Reaven [1] suggested that resistance to insulin and hyperinsulinemia are involved in the etiology and natural history of three major diseases, namely non-insulin-dependent diabetes (NIDDM), essential hypertension and ischemic heart disease. He proposed the name of syndrome X for a cluster of variables that tend to occur in the same individual. These variables include insulin resistance to insulin-stimulated glucose uptake, glucose intolerance or NIDDM, hyperinsulinemia, increased very low density lipoprotein (VLDL) triglycerides, decreased high density lipoprotein (HDL) cholesterol and essential hypertension. While central obesity was not mentioned in the initial description, there is evidence to suggest that this phenotype should be included as part of this syndrome [2].

Syndrome X and the links between insulin resistance, hyperinsulinemia and hypertension became rapidly very popular. Numerous studies, many symposia, reviews and newspaper special issues have been devoted to this up-to-date topic, most of them being supported by pharma-

Philippe Passa
Department of Endocrinology and Diabetology
Hospital Saint-Louis
1, av. Claude-Vellefaux
F–75010 Paris (France)

0301–0163/92/0382–0033
$2.75/0

ceutical companies. At the present time, all the physicians concerned with prevention and treatment of cardiovascular diseases have to be aware of the current knowledge about this fascinating story. Syndrome X may be a very important topic, supporting the concept that essential hypertension is a metabolic disorder [3] and giving an explanation to the current failure of coronary artery disease (CAD) prevention [4]. On the other hand, many issues are still to be solved, many aspects are still controversial and from a scientific point of view the end of the story is still unknown.

It must be emphasized that the story started a long time ago. In 1956, Prof. Jean Vague [5] reported that central obesity was associated with a cluster of metabolic disorders, risk factors for atherosclerosis. Thirteen years ago, three major epidemiological prospective studies conducted in Australia [6], Finland [7] and France [8] reported concordant data, cardiovascular mortality was independently associated with fasting plasma insulin values and/or insulinemia 2 h after oral glucose load.

Hyperinsulinemia and Essential Hypertension

Hyperinsulinemia as a link between hypertension, obesity and glucose intolerance was reported for the first time by Modan et al. [9] in 1985. Hypertension and glucose intolerance determined in a random population sample from Israel (n = 2,475) showed a highly significant association from the mildest levels of both conditions, independent of the confounding variables. Fasting and post-glucose load insulin levels, in a representative subgroup, were significantly elevated in hypertensive subjects, independently of obesity, glucose intolerance, age and antihypertensive medications. The mean increment in summed 1- and 2-hour insulin levels (mU/l) compared with non-obese normotensives with normal glucose tolerance, was 12 for hypertension alone, 47 for obesity alone, 52 for impaired glucose tolerance and 124 when all three conditions were present. The conclusion was reached that hypertension per se is associated with hyperinsulinemia and this can be thought of as one common ground for the clustering of diabetes, obesity and essential hypertension.

In a large group of subjects with impaired glucose tolerance, Christlieb et al. [10] found higher serum insulin levels in those subjects who had diastolic hypertension in comparison with those with systolic hypertension or normal blood pressure. In a bi-ethnic population of nondiabetic Mexican-Americans and non-Hispanic Whites, the sum of insulin values after an oral glucose load was directly related to both systolic and diastolic blood pressure in men, after accounting for degree of obesity and body fat distribution [11]. These previous studies have been repeatedly confirmed and it is now clearly demonstrated that essential hypertension is associated with hyperinsulinemia.

Hypertension and Insulin Resistance

What is the reason for the hyperinsulinemia in subjects with essential hypertension? It is now well known that both obesity [12] and NIDDM [13] are characterized by insulin resistance. In the broad sense of the word, insulin resistance is defined by a reduced, impaired or different response of target tissues to insulin stimulation. Although it is customary to refer insulin action to glucose metabolism, it should be kept in mind that any of the actions of insulin on carbohydrate, fat, protein and electrolyte metabolism can be impaired and that a defect in one insulin action does not imply that other actions of insulin are equally affected. In nondiabetic patients with hypertension compared to normotensive control subjects it has been shown by Singer et al. [14] that diurnal fasting and postprandial plasma insulin levels were significantly higher in spite of similar levels of plasma glucose. These data suggested that hypertension is an insulin-resistant state. The existence of insulin resistance in essential hypertensive patients was also suggested and then demonstrated by Ferrannini and co-workers [15] in a series of elegant studies. In nondiabetic hypertensive subjects of either sex with mild degrees of obesity, the insulin response to oral glucose was significantly heightened in comparison with age-, sex- and weight-matched normotensive subjects. Furthermore, in the hypertensive group there was a strong relationship between the 2-hour plasma insulin level and blood pressure. To avoid the confounding influence of obesity and impaired glucose tolerance, the same group also carried out oral glucose tolerance tests in young, nonobese, hypertensives of both sexes with normal glucose tolerance. In comparison with age- and weight-matched normotensive subjects, the hypertensive patients exhibited higher plasma insulin levels at all times following glucose ingestion. It is to be noted that although within the normal range by conventional diagnostic criteria, plasma glucose levels were also higher in the hypertensives than in controls during the second hour of the test [16]. In the same group of hypertensive patients, Ferrannini et al. [16] have measured several actions of insulin in vivo, using rather refined and reliable techniques: euglycemic hyperinsulinemic clamp technique, glucose tracer infusions and indirect calorimetry. The results obtained showed that: (a) hypertensives as a mean utilized 40% less glucose than matched normotensives in response to a physiological increment in plasma insulin levels; however, important individual variations were to be noticed; (b) the ability of insulin to suppress hepatic glucose production was preserved; (c) only nonoxidative glucose disposal partakes in the reduction in total glucose metabolism, glucose oxidation being unaltered, and (d) effects of insulin on potassium uptake and lipolysis were normal. The decrease in insulin glucose uptake was directly related to the degree of systolic hypertension. From this study it is possible to conclude that essential hypertension (independently of body weight and glucose tolerance) is associated with an insulin resistance that is apparently primary, peripheral in location and metabolically selective. These characteristics are different to those observed in insulin resistance associated with obesity or NIDDM, so the underlying causes must be, at least in part, different.

Role of Insulin Resistance and Hyperinsulinemia in Pathogenesis of Hypertension

The correlations between hyperinsulinemia, insulin resistance and blood pressure values do not prove that the relationship is a causal one. However, if one postulates that insulin resistance and hyperinsulinemia are involved in the etiology of hypertension, it is possible to find data, both in animal models and in humans, that provide support for this hypothesis.

In two unrelated animal models of hypertension, spontaneously hypertensive rats (SHR) and in Dahl rats, Reaven et al. [17] have documented the presence of lipid changes, hyperinsulinemia and reduced insulin-mediated glucose uptake by adipocytes in vitro. In Sprague-Dawley rats, the impairment of insulin-mediated glucose uptake precedes the appearance of hypertension. Similar changes in glucose, insulin metabolism and blood pressure can be experimentally produced also in normal and Sprague-Dawley rats, when feeding them high fructose diets [18]. These effects of fructose can be prevented by exercise training [19] or somatostatin [20]. However, it should be mentioned that neither SHR nor Dahl rats have been found to be insulin-resistant in vivo during euglycemic hyperinsulinemia.

In humans, it has been shown that weight reduction improves insulin sensitivity, reduces hyperinsulinemia and blood pressure [21]. In a similar fashion, the decline in blood pressure associated with exercise training seems to be limited to individuals who were initially hyperinsulinemic and had the greatest fall in plasma insulin level as a result of the training program [22]. Finally, in the San Antonio Heart Study, hyperinsulinemia in nondiabetic offsprings of diabetic parents was associated with a higher prevalence of hypertension. Subclinical changes in glucose tolerance, lipid levels and insulin concentrations coexisted with slight elevations in both systolic and diastolic blood pressure in healthy subjects, 8 years before hypertension developed [23]. To be fair, it must be mentioned that different data are not in keeping with a causal relation between hyperinsulinemia and hypertension.

To determine whether chronic hyperinsulinemia comparable to that found in obesity-associated hypertension may modify blood pressure, Hall et al. [24] infused insulin with glucose in experimental dogs. For 7–28 days, raised plasma insulin by 5- to 10-fold did not significantly change mean arterial pressure in dogs with reduced kidney mass that were maintained on high sodium diet. In dogs infused with angiotensin II, to raise mild hypertension, insulin infusion for 28 days did not potentiate the hypertension. In humans, patients with insulinomas do not present with increased blood pressure; after surgical removal, the dramatic reduction in plasma insulin levels is not associated with a decrease in blood pressure [25].

Metformin, an oral antidiabetic agent whose mechanism of action is primarily an improvement in insulin sensitivity, has been extensively used in NIDDM, at least in France, for nearly 40 years. It has never been reported by a French group that this drug could modify blood pressure in normotensive or hypertensive NIDDM diabetic patients. However, Landin et al. [26] during a short-term, uncontrolled study in a small group of hypertensive patients reported a significant antihypertensive effect of metformin. In insulin-dependent and in insulin-requiring diabetic patients, exogenous insulin administration results in frank hyperinsulinemia. It has not been commonly reported that such patients may suffer high prevalence of essential hypertension (in the absence of diabetic kidney disease). Although in a small group of NIDDM women taking insulin doses over their needs, insulin dosage reduction was associated with a decrease in blood pressure in hypertensives; no modification in blood pressure occurred in normotensives [27]. So from the available data, the direct causal role of hyperinsulinemia in essential hypertension is still to be proved, at least in humans. Great care should be exercised in the extrapolation of results of studies in rats or dogs to hypertensive humans.

Whatever the real role is, hyperinsulinemia could increase blood pressure by different mechanisms, and has recently been reviewed by De Fronzo and Ferrannini [28, 29]. In the present paper, the data dealing with the potential hypertensive effects of insulin will be briefly summarized.

Hyperinsulinemia could raise blood pressure by increasing sodium reabsorption at the level of the renal tubule. In healthy subjects, acute physiological hyperinsulinemia with maintenance of euglycemia decreases urinary sodium excretion thereby promoting sodium retention. There is, however, no change in blood pressure whilst using the euglycemic clamp technique with physiological insulin doses. Nevertheless, it is conceivable that chronic elevations of insulin concentrations might lead to an increase in the body sodium content and an abnormal sensitivity to pressive hormones [30]. A second mechanism by which insulin can cause hypertension involves stimulation of the sympathetic nervous system (SNS). Numerous studies in animals and humans have shown that insulin activates the SNS and this in turn may promote hypertension through various mechanisms: increased cardiac output, peripheral vasoconstriction [for review, see 31]. Insulin may also disturb Na^+ and H^+ pump activity [32]. The intracellular accumulation of Na^+ and Ca^{2+} would be expected to enhance the sensitivity of the vascular smooth musculature to the pressor effects of norepinephrine, angiotensin and NaCl loading. Finally, insulin acting directly or indirectly through the stimulation of growth factors, such as IGF-1, may also contribute to the development of hypertension by causing hypertrophy of the vascular wall and the narrowing of the lumen of the resistance vessels involved in the regulation of systemic blood pressure [33].

In conclusion, many data support the hypothesis that hyperinsulinemia may play a central causal role in the development of essential hypertension in several insulin-resistant states; however, for the time being the definite demonstration of such a role is still lacking.

Hyperinsulinemia and Antihypertensive Treatment

Drug therapy has improved the prognosis of hypertension with a decrease in mortality having been observed in severe, moderate and mild hypertension. This overall improvement has been due to a reduction in mortality from cardiac failure, renal failure and cerebrovascular accidents. In general, the reduction in mortality from CAD has been less impressive.

Three studies have not shown any significant change in mortality from CAD [34–36]. One demonstrated a significant beneficial effect in a population of hypertensives over 65 years of age [37]. Although the reason (or reasons) for this failure is unknown, various suggestions have been proposed. Amongst them, one is related to the metabolic undesirable side effects of the antihypertensive drugs used in these trials: diuretics and β-blockers. Both types of drug may alter lipoprotein profile [38, 39] and such an alteration may increase the risk of atherosclerosis and CAD. Diuretics and β-blockers may also modify glucose metabolism. Studies from Scandinavia have suggested that the occurrence of hypertension and NIDDM in the same patient may be partly due to antihypertensive therapy [40–42]. In each of these longitudinal studies, the development of hypertension tended to precede that of NIDDM at a much greater frequency that could be explained by chance. Skarfors et al. [41] were also able to show that treated hypertensive patients had hyperinsulinemia, decreased insulin sensitivity, higher serum triglycerides, and lower HDL cholesterol levels when compared with matched controls or untreated hypertensives [41]. Over the past few years, Pollare et al. [43, 44] have investigated the effects of antihypertensive agents on insulin resistance, using the euglycemic insulin clamp technique. In a series of studies, they have shown that representative drugs of two classes – angiotensin-converting enzyme inhibitors (captopril) and selective peripheral α_1-blockers (prazosin) – improve insulin sensitivity in hypertensive individuals. The calcium entry blocker (diltiazem) did not affect insulin sensitivity [45], whereas the β-blockers (metoprolol and atenolol) [46] and thiazide diuretics (hydrochlorothiazide) [43] both worsened insulin sensitivity. As would be anticipated, decreased insulin sensitivity was associated with an increase in serum triglycerides. Whether differences regarding insulin resistance exist between antihypertensive drugs from the same class, is still controversial and currently under investigation. For ACE inhibitors, in our group, we did not observe any influence of enalapril on insulin sensitivity in normotensive or hypertensive IDDM patients [47].

The data from the studies we reviewed suggest that calcium entry blockers and ACE inhibitors, which do not have undesirable metabolic side effects, should be selected as drug of choice in patients with essential hypertension. However, it must be recalled, firstly, that many other criteria apart from insulin sensitivity are to be taken into account for the choice of an antihypertensive agent, and secondly that these new classes of antihypertensive agents have not been tested in long-term prospective clinical trials; thus we do not yet know if they would reduce mortality and morbidity as well as or better than older antihypertensive agents.

Conclusion

There are many arguments to suggest that hyperinsulinemia (cause or consequence of insulin resistance) may play a key role in the natural history of essential hypertension and in the metabolic disorders and cardiovascular complications commonly associated with this condition. Furthermore, the presence of hyperinsulinemia and insulin resistance in subjects with asymptomatic atherosclerosis, but with normal weight, glucose tolerance, blood pressure and serum lipid levels, has been recently demonstrated [48]. To prevent ischemic vascular disease, hyperinsulinemia should be corrected early in life. We still do ignore if such an attitude will be feasible and effective. The end of the syndrome X story will be known when the data of long-term prospective epidemiological, clinical and genetical studies become available.

References

1 Reaven GM: Role of insulin resistance in human disease. Diabetes 1988;37:1595–1607.
2 Bjorntorp P: The associations between obesity, adipose tissue and disease. Acta Med Scand 1988(suppl 723):121–134.
3 Ferrannini E: Metabolic abnormalities of hypertension. A lesson in complexity. Hypertension 1991;18:636–639.
4 Black HR: The coronary artery disease paradox: The role for hyperinsulinemia and insulin resistance, implications for therapy. J Cardiovasc Pharmacol 1990;15(suppl 5):S26–S38.
5 Vague J: The degree of masculine differentiation of obesities, a factor determining predisposition to diabetes, atherosclerosis, gout and uric calculous diseases. Am J Clin Nutr 1956;4:20–34.
6 Welborn TA, Wearne K: Coronary heart disease incidence and cardiovascular mortality in Busselton with reference to glucose and insulin concentrations. Diabetes Care 1979;2:154–160.
7 Pyörälä K: Relationship of glucose tolerance and plasma insulin to the incidence of coronary heart disease, results from two population studies in Finland. Diabetes Care 1979;2:131–141.
8 Ducimetiere P, Eschwege E, Papoz L, Richard JL, Claude JR, Rosselin GE: Relationship of plasma insulin levels to the incidence of myocardial infarction and coronary heart disease in a middle-aged population. Diabetologia 1980;19:205–210.
9 Modan M, Halkin H, Almog S, et al: Hyperinsulinemia, a link between hypertension, obesity and glucose intolerance. J Clin Invest 1985;75:809–817.
10 Christlieb AR, Krolewski AS, Warram JH, Soeldner JS: Is insulin the link between hypertension and obesity? Hypertension 1985;7(suppl II):54–57.
11 Haffner SM, Fong D, Hazuda HP, Pugh JA, Patterson JK: Hyperinsulinemia, upper body adiposity and cardiovascular risk factors in non-diabetics. Metabolism 1988;37:338–345.
12 Olefsky JM, Kolterman OG, Scarlett JA: Insulin action and resistance in obesity and non-insulin-dependent (type II) diabetes mellitus. Am J Physiol 1982;243:15–30.
13 Bogardus C, Lillioja S, Howard B, Reaven GM, Mott D: Relationships between insulin secretion, insulin action and fasting plasma glucose concentration in non-diabetic and non-insulin-dependent diabetic subjects. J Clin Invest 1984;74:1238–1246.
14 Singer P, Godicke W, Voigt S, Hadju I, Weiss M: Postprandial hyperinsulinemia in patients with mild hypertension. Hypertension 1985;7:182–186.
15 Manicardi V, Camellini L, Bellodi G, Coscelli C, Ferrannini E: Evidence for an association of high blood pressure and hyperinsulinemia in obese man. J Clin Endocrinol Metab 1986;62:1302–1304.
16 Ferrannini E, Buzzigoli G, Bonadonna R, et al: Insulin resistance in essential hypertension. N Engl J Med 1987;317:350–357.
17 Reaven GM, Chang H, Hoffman BB, Azmar S: Resistance to insulin-stimulated glucose uptake in adipocytes isolated from spontaneously hypertensive rats. Diabetes 1989;38:1155–1160.
18 Huang IS, Ho H, Hoffman BB, Reaven GM: Fructose-induced insulin resistance and hypertension in rats. Hypertension 1987;10:512–516.
19 Reaven GM, Ho H, Hoffman BB: Attenuation of fructose-induced hypertension in rats by exercise training. Hypertension 1988;12:129–132.
20 Reaven GM, Ho H, Hoffman BB: Somatostatin inhibition of fructose-induced hypertension. Hypertension 1989;14:117–120.
21 Reisin E, Abel R, Modan M, Silverberg DS, Eliahou HE, Modan B: Effect of weight loss without salt restriction on the reduction of blood pressure in overweight hypertensive patients. N Engl J Med 1978;298:1–6.
22 Krotielowski M, Mandroukas K, Sjostrom L, Sullivan L, Wetterauist H, Bjorntorp P: Effects of long-term physical training on body fast, metabolism and blood pressure in obesity. Metabolism 1979;28:650–658.
23 Haffner SM, Stern MP, Hazuda HP, Mitchell BD, Patterson JK, Ferrannini E: Parental history of diabetes is associated with increased cardiovascular risk factors. Arteriosclerosis 1989;9:928–933.
24 Hall JE, Coleman TG, Mizelle HL: Does chronic hyperinsulinemia cause hypertension? Am J Hypertens 1989;2:171–173.
25 Tsutsu N, Nunoi K, Kodama T, Nomiyama R, Iwase M, Fujishima M: Lack of association between blood pressure and insulin in patients with insulinoma. J Hypertens 1990;8:479–482.
26 Landin K, Tengborn L, Smith U: Treating insulin resistance in hypertension with metformin reduces both blood pressure and metabolic risk factors. J Intern Med 1991;229:181–187.
27 Tedde R, Sechi LA, Marigliano A, Pala A, Scano L: Antihypertensive effect of insulin reduction in diabetic hypertensive patients. Am J Hypertens 1989;2:163–170.
28 Ferrannini E, De Fronzo RA: The association of hypertension, diabetes and obesity: A review. J Nephrol 1989;1:3–15.
29 De Fronzo RA, Ferrannini E: Insulin resistance: A multifaceted syndrome responsible for NIDDM, obesity, hypertension, dyslipidemia and atherosclerotic cardiovascular disease. Diabetes Care 1991;14:173–194.
30 Weidmann P, Ferrari P: Central role of sodium in hypertension in diabetic subjects. Diabetes Care 1991;14:220–232.
31 Modan M, Halkin H: Hyperinsulinemia or increased sympathetic drive as links for obesity and hypertension. Diabetes Care 1991;14:470–487.
32 Huot SJ, Aronson PS: Na^+-H^+ exchange and its role in essential hypertension and diabetes mellitus. Diabetes Care 1991;14:521–535.

33 Mulvany MJ: Pathophysiology of vascular smooth muscle in hypertension. J Hypertens 1984;2(suppl III): 413–420.
34 Australian National Blood Pressure Study Management Committee: The Australian therapeutic trial in mild hypertension. Lancet 1980;i:1261–1267.
35 Medical Research Council Working Party: MRC trial of treatment of mild hypertension: Principal results. Br Med J 1985;291:97–104.
36 Hypertension Detection and Follow-Up Program Cooperative Group: Five-year findings of the hypertension detection and follow-up program. I Reduction in mortality of persons with high blood pressure, including mild hypertension. JAMA 1979;242:2562–2571.
37 Amery A, Birkenhager W, Briyko P, et al: Mortality and morbidity results from European working party on high blood pressure in the elderly trial. Lancet 1985;i:1349–1354.
38 Ames RP: Negative effects of diuretic drugs on metabolic risk factors for coronary heart disease: Possible alternative drug therapies. Am J Cardiol 1983;51:632–638.
39 Weinberger MH: Antihypertensive therapy and lipids: Evidence, mechanisms and implications. Arch Intern Med 1985;145:1102–1105.
40 Bengtsson C, Blohme G, Lapidus L, et al: Do antihypertensive drugs precipitate diabetes? Br Med J 1984;289:1495–1497.
41 Skarfors ET, Lithell HO, Selinus I, Aberg H: Do antihypertensive drugs precipitate diabetes in predisposed men? Br Med J 1989;298:1147–1152.
42 Lundgren H, Bjorkman L, Keiding P, Lundmark S, Bengtsson C: Diabetes in patients with hypertension receiving pharmacological treatment. Br Med J 1988;297:1512.
43 Pollare T, Lithell H, Berne C: A comparison of the effects of hydrochlorothiazide and captopril on glucose and lipid metabolism in patients with hypertension. N Engl J Med 1989; 321:868–873.
44 Pollare T, Lithell H, Selinus I, Berne C: Application of prazosin is associated with an increase of insulin sensitivity in obese patients with hypertension. Diabetologia 1988;31:415–420.
45 Pollare T, Lithell H, Morlin C, Prantare H, Huarfner A, Ljunghall S: Metabolism effects of diltiazem and atenolol: Results from a randomized, double-blind study with parallel groups. J Hypertens 1989;7:551–559.
46 Pollare T, Lithell H, Selinus I, Berne C: Sensitivity to insulin during treatment with atenolol and metoprolol: A randomized double-blind study of effects on carbohydrate and lipoprotein metabolism in hypertensive patients. Br Med J 1989;298:1152–1157.
47 Leblanc H, Thote A, Billault B, Porquet D, Fisch A, Passa Ph: Absence d'effet de l'enalapril sur le contrôle glycémique et la sensibilité à l'insuline chez 10 diabétiques insulino-dépendants traités par infusion continue sous-cutanée d'insuline. Presse Méd 1988;43:2277–2280.
48 Laakso M, Sarlund H, Salonen R, Suhoneu M, Pyörälä K, Salonen JT, Karhapää P: Asymptomatic atherosclerosis and insulin resistance. Arterioscler Thromb 1991;11:1068–1076.

Horm Res 1992;38:39–40

François Berthezene

Service d'Endocrinologie et des Maladies de la Nutrition, INSERM U. 63, Hôpital de l'Antiquaille, Lyon, France

Hypertriglyceridemia: Cause or Consequence of Insulin Resistance?

Key Words
Hypertriglyceridemia
Diabetes
Insulin resistance
Free fatty acids

Abstract
An overproduction of VLDL by the liver and a slower clearance of these lipoproteins are usually seen in diabetic patients. There is correlation between insulin resistance and plasma triglyceride concentration. Triglyceride may influence an early step in the insulin action pathway and alternatively, insulin resistance may cause hypertriglyceridemia. Hyperinsulinemia and/or hypertriglyceridemia may play a strong role in the cardiovascular risk of patients with type II diabetes. There is an important need to conduct trials to define therapy that can reduce the risk of cadiovascular complications.

The most common alteration of lipoproteins in type II diabetes is an increase in triglyceride concentration. There is an overproduction of VLDL by the liver and a slower clearance of these lipoproteins [1]. The VLDL composition is changed in patients with type II diabetes; these particles are large, triglyceride-rich with an increase in triglyceride/Apo B ratio. Kinetic studies have shown that large VLDL are less efficiently converted to LDL [2].

Significant correlations exist beween insulin resistance, as measured by the euglycemic clamp technique, and plasma triglyceride concentration [1, 3, 4]. Experimental manipulations which modify insulin action have led to predictable changes in triglyceride concentration; weight loss and exercise are both associated with a large decrease in plasma insulin and triglyceride concentration.

The mechanisms for the overproduction and the decrease in metabolic clearance rate of VLDL and their relationship with insulin resistance are not clear. Several studies have investigated the effects of lipid-lowering agents on glucose tolerance in patients with type II diabetes. Bezafibrate, a fibric acid derivative, which lowers free fatty acid and triglyceride concentrations, decreases fasting glycemia, insulin and C-peptide levels [5] suggesting a role of lipids on glucose tolerance. In contrast, nicotinic acid administration which improves lipoprotein profile, chiefly plasma triglyceride levels, in patients with type II diabetes, results in the deterioration of glycemic control [6, 7]. Plasma triglycerides may influence early steps in the insulin action pathway such as insulin receptor binding, but after normalization of triglyceride levels, improvement in insulin binding does not occur [8]. There is a strong negative correlation between muscle triglyceride and potency of insulin action [9]; a buildup of lipid in muscle would lead to insulin resistance via the glucose-fatty acid cycle. In fact, plasma free fatty acids and not triglyceride concentration may be of importance for the

François Berthezene
Service d'Endocrinologie et des Maladies de la Nutrition
INSERM U. 63
Hôpital de l'Antiquaille
F–69321 Lyon (France)

0301–0163/92/0382–0039
$2.75/0

development of insulin resistance. Antilipolytic agents improve insulin action in diabetic patients [10] and free fatty acids can inhibit insulin-stimulated glucose uptake and impair insulin binding to hepatocytes [11].

Alternatively, insulin resistance may cause hypertriglyceridemia. Metformin, a biguanide which ameliorates insulin resistance, may decrease in patients with type II diabetes VLDL triglyceride levels [12]. Insulin resistance may decrease adipose tissue but not skeletal muscle lipoprotein lipase activity [1] and so restrain removal of triglyceride-rich particles. Muscle tissue is a more important site for triglyceride hydrolysis than adipose tissue [2] and it is not evident that the effect of insulin resistance on lipoprotein lipase activity plays an important role in hypertriglyceridemic patients. The removal defect of VLDL is more likely due to the changes of VLDL composition [2]. Insulin resistance may induce an increase in secretion of triglycerides by the liver either directly or by an increase in glucose and free fatty acid plasma concentrations. The elevation in VLDL production in patients with type II diabetes is more likely due to the increase in free fatty acid production seen in these patients. Studies with perfused liver and hepatocytes have shown that fatty acids have a stimulatory effect on the synthesis and secretion of VLDL triglycerides; in contrast, insulin causes a decrease in the secretion of triglycerides [13]. The fasting free fatty acid concentration is on the average similar in hyper- and normotriglyceridemic patients but, in hypertriglyceridemic diabetic patients, there is a defect in postprandial or insulin suppression of free fatty acid [14]; this is characteristic of hypertriglyceridemia seen in patients with type II diabetes.

Cardiovascular disease is the principal cause of morbidity and mortality in patients with type II diabetes. Hypertriglyceridmia may play a strong role in the cardiovascular risk of these patients but no clinical trial has tested the efficacy of treatments on cardiovascular complications. Several studies have demonstrated that glycemic control with biguanides, sulfonylureas or insulin can improve diabetic dyslipidemia [7]. Abdominal obesity is very closley linked to insulin resistance. The most likely explanation is that triglyceride mobilization is high in visceral fat; a large output of free fatty acid into the portal vein has several effects on the liver leading to hyperglycemia and hypertriglyceridemia [15]. Reduction of abdominal obesity by diet and exercice produces favorable changes in diabetic dyslipidemia. Lipid-lowering agents, chiefly fibrates and presumably HMG-CoA reductase inhibitors, may be of value in the treatment of diabetic dyslipidemia. There is an important need to conduct trials in patients with type II diabetes to define the optimum regimen and the therapy that can reduce the risk of cardiovascular complications.

References

1 Howard BV: Lipoprotein metabolism in diabetes mellitus. J Lipid Res 1987;28:613–628.
2 Taskinen MJ, Packard CJ, Shepherd J: Effect of insulin therapy on metabolic fat of apolipoprotein B-containing lipoproteins in NIDDM. Diabetes 1990;39:1017–1027.
3 Reaven GM: Resistance to insulin-stimulated glucose uptake and hyperinsulinemia: Role in non-insulin-dependent diabetes, high blood pressure, dyslipidemia and coronary heart disease. Diabete Metab 1991;17:78–86.
4 Abbott WGH, Lillioja S, Young AA, Zawadzki JK, Yki-Järvinen H, Christin L, Howard BV: Relationships between plasma lipoprotein concentrations and insulin action in an obese hyperinsulinemic population. Diabetes 1987;36: 897–904.
5 Jones IR, Swai A, Taylor R, Miller M, Laker MF, Alberti KGMM: Lowering of plasma glucose concentrations with bezafibrate in patients with moderately controlled NIDDM. Diabetes Care 1990;13:855–863.
6 Garg A, Grundy SM: Nicotinic acid as therapy for dyslipidemia in non-insulin-dependent diabetes mellitus. JAMA 1990;264:723–726.
7 Stern MP, Haffner SM: Dyslipidemia in type II diabetes. Implications for therapeutic intervention. Diabetes Care 1991;14:1144–1159.
8 Cordera R, Bertolini S, Andraghetti G, Pistocchi G, De Alessi M, Gherzi R: Insulin receptor binding on red cells of hypertriglyceridemic patients. Effect of a low fat, low carbohydrate diet. Diabete Metab 1985;11:137–140.
9 Kraegen EW, Clark PW, Jenkins AB, Daley EA, Chisholm DJ, Storlien LH: Development of muscle insulin resistance after liver insulin resistance in high fat fed rats. Diabetes 1991; 40:1397–1403.
10 Vaag A, Skött P, Damsbo P, Gall M-A, Richter EA, Beck-Nielsen H: Effect of the antilipolytic nicotinic acid analogue acipimox on whole-body and skeletal muscle glucose metabolism in patients with non-insulin-dependent diabetes mellitus. J Clin Invest 1991;88:1282–1290.
11 Svedberg J, Björntorp P, Smith U, Lönnroth P: Effect of free fatty acids on insulin receptor binding and tyrosine kinase activity in hepatocytes isolated from lean and obese rats. Diabetes 1992;41:294–298.
12 Schneider J: Effects of metformin on dyslipoproteinemia in non-insulin-dependent diabetes mellitus. Diabete Metab 1991;17:185–190.
13 Dashti N, Wolfbauer G: Secretion of lipids, apolipoproteins, and lipoproteins by human hepatoma cell line Hep G2: Effects of oleic acid and insulin. J Lipid Res 1987;28:423–436.
14 Yki-Järvinen H, Taskinen M-R: Interrelationships among insulin's antilipolytic and glucoregulatory effects and plasma triglycerides in nondiabetic and diabetic patients with endogenous hypertriglyceridemia. Diabetes 1988;37: 1271–1277.
15 Björntorp P: New concepts in the relationship obesity-non-insulin dependent diabetes mellitus. Prog Med 1992;1:37–41.

Horm Res 1992;38:41–45

D. Dewailly
C. Cortet-Rudelli

Service d'Endocrinologie et de Diabétologie, USN A-CHRU de Lille, France

Insulin Resistance and Polycystic Ovarian Syndrome

Key Words
Insulin
Hyperandrogenism
Polycystic ovarian syndrome
Puberty
Insulin-like growth factor

Abstract
Insulin resistance (IR) and polycystic ovarian syndrome (PCOS) appear as linked phenomena, although this is not easy to obviate in common forms of PCOS while it is evident in the rare cases of extreme IR and hyperinsulinism (HI). Experimental data indicate that insulin could interfere with the local insulin-like growth factor systems in ovaries, and presumably in adrenals and in the hypothalamic pituitary system. The female puberty system offers a physiological model to explain the gonadotropic action of insulin. In patients with IR, HI could induce a state of hyperpuberty, leading to the constitution of PCOS during adolescence.

Introduction

The polycystic ovary syndrome (PCOS) is a complex functional and morphological disorder which affects a great proportion of young women. Its main clinical features, i.e. hyperandrogenism and infertility, are the consequences of an excessive stimulation of the theca-interstitial cells and of an impairment in the development of granulosa cells, respectively. The former abnormality can be explained by an excessive production and/or action of LH while the latter is considered to be the consequence of an impaired production and/or action of FSH. Therefore, the hypothalamic-pituitary system is placed by most authors at the center of the physiopathogenic scheme of PCOS.

However, other factors are thought to be involved and the role of insulin has been highlighted these recent years. The peculiar involvement of a pancreatic hormone in the ovarian physiology and pathology was first suspected from clinical observations with severe hyperinsulinism (HI) due to an insulin resistance (IR), and then detailed by experimental data. Nevertheless, many points remain obscure, although very recent studies give an insight into the crucial role that insulin may play via its interaction with the growth factors [1].

Clinical Data

That a pathological HI is able to stimulate the androgen secretion from the ovaries was the conclusion of a debate in the literature about clinical cases of severe IR, within the frame of the HAIR syndromes [2]. It is not the point of this review to recall the numerous arguments in

D. Dewailly
Service d'Endocrinologie et de Diabétologie
USN A-CHRU de Lille
F-59000 Lille (France)

0301–0163/92/0382–0041
$2.75/0

favor of the following sequency: IR → HI → hyperandrogenism [3, 4]. In these rare instances, plasma insulin levels are 10- to 100-fold those of normal subjects, thus reflecting a severe IR due to either receptor or postreceptor defects whose molecular characteristics are described in the current literature [5, 6]. The hyperandrogenism is the consequence of a severe PCOS which sometimes borders on hyperthecosis. It may be lessened by therapeutical means aiming at reducing the endogenous LH levels [7].

Apart from these exceptional clinical observations, a mild IR is also suspected in some women with more common forms of PCOS. However, the literature available at the present time is somewhat flawed by data collected in nonrepresentative groups of patients with PCOS. Some included a high proportion of women with obesity and/or acanthosis nigricans, whose frequencies in a large cohort of patients with PCOS are only 30 and 4%, respectively. Therefore, one might assume that some patients included in these studies were in fact moderate HAIR syndromes. Nevertheless, these data suggest that a mild to medium HI was directly involved in the hyperandrogenism, since significant positive correlations were found between plasma insulin and androgen levels [8–11]. However, the exact prevalence of HI (and therefore IR) within the whole spectrum of PCOS remains to be evaluated.

More recent studies attempted to address this issue in nonselected women in whom PCOS was ascertained by ultrasound. No precise evaluation of the prevalence of IR in PCOS can be drawn at the present time, due to the heterogeneity of clinical presentation of patients from one study to the other, and to the different criteria used to detect IR. By using a fasting plasma insulin level > mean of controls + 2 SD, Conway et al. [12] found that 30% of patients with PCOS had a mild IR, although no one was overweight in this series. With the minimum model analysis, Falcone et al. [13] found that 63% of their patients were insulin-resistant. In our own experience [12], 29% of our patients had an excessive insulin response during OGTT. The main flaw of these studies is that a not sufficiently large general population of women was investigated in parallel with the patients. Therefore, it is still not possible to claim that IR is really more frequent in PCOS than in the general population.

Furthermore, several groups recently reported that no correlation between plasma insulin and androgen levels could be found in more representative groups of patients than those included in the previous studies [12, 14–16]. Therefore, one could conclude from these data that HI is not determinant in common forms of PCOS and that its role is restricted to the severely insulin-resistant patients. However, two studies have recently reinforced the pathogenic role of insulin by showing that reduction of HI, either by diazoxide [17] or low caloric diet [18], improves some clinical [18] and hormonal [17, 18] abnormalities of the common forms of PCOS. On the other hand, acute stimulation of insulin secretion in the aim to stimulate ovarian androgens leads to conflicting results in the literature, mainly for technical reasons [1]. Although no definitive conclusion can be drawn at the present time, it can be summarized from clinical data that insulin resistance is probably an important part of the physiopathology of PCOS but this is difficult to obviate in clinical practice. This is mainly explained by the lack of sensitivity and reproducibility of the available criteria of IR used in clinical studies. It could also be explained by the fact that most women are investigated at a period of life when the relationships between insulin and ovaries are not the closest. This will be discussed later.

Experimental Data

It is now well established that the ovary has insulin receptors as well as type 1 insulin-like growth factor (IGF) receptors, both hormone and receptor structures sharing a relative homology [19]. It has been already fully discussed how insulin may act on ovarian cells despite the state of IR [19]. According to cell culture data, insulin mimics the effects of IGF-1 both on granulosa and theca-interstitial cells and may therefore alter the condition of the paracrine events occurring in the ovarian follicles which are under the dependence of IGFs [20]. Direct stimulating effects of insulin and IGF-1 on theca-interstitial cells, and thus on androgen synthesis, have been reported, although the insulin concentrations in medium have to be supraphysiological while the effective concentrations of IGF-1 are within the physiological range [21]. Furthermore, the presence of LH and FSH is required and the only relevant effects of insulin and IGF-1 are in fact to amplify the local action of these gonadotropins [22].

Therefore, there is still a missing link between the in vivo and in vitro data since the degree of HI in patients with PCOS is not high enough to allow insulin plasma levels to directly stimulate the theca-interstitial cells, even in the presence of high plasma LH levels. Furthermore, there is at yet no evidence that insulin enhances the local production of IGF-1 by ovarian cells.

Attempting a Unifying Concept

To try to improve our understanding of the involvement of insulin in PCOS, it is necessary to refer to physiological models, and especially to female puberty and growth [23].

At the ovarian levels, the early changes occurring at puberty are induced by the combined actions of gonadotropins and local growth factors. Very recent animal data [24] showed that IGF-1 and its type 1 receptor are maximally expressed during the peripubertal period. From cell culture data it is known that IGF-1 is able to enhance DNA synthesis by both types of ovarian follicular cells from many species, including humans [25]. Likewise, it stimulates some key enzymes such as FSH-dependent aromatase in granulosa cells and LH-dependent cytochrome P-450 c17 in theca-interstitial cells [26]. Therefore, it is tempting to speculate that IGF-1 is an important factor of pubertal ovarian development, although it is not proven that its presence is absolutely necessary. Similar findings have been reported in adrenals, where IGF-1 appears to stimulate the effects of ACTH in cultured adrenal cells [27]. Although no evidence for this has been reported yet, one might speculate that IGF-1 plays a role in pubertal adrenal maturation, which is accompanied by the increase of some enzymatic activities, such as the cytochrome P-450 c17 [28].

At least for ovarian tissues, insulin has been shown to mimic the effects of IGF-1 under experimental conditions [21, 22, 26]. On the other hand, the effects of insulin on adrenal function are less documented, although some data suggest that it could physiologically inhibit the 17,20-lyase activity [29]. However, no direct evidence is available to date, meaning that insulin could interfere in vivo with the pubertal maturation of ovaries, adrenals and the hypothalamic pituitary system. In contrast, a strong inverse relationship has been found in physiologic and pathologic conditions between insulin and two plasma proteins which are produced by the liver and which play a key role in the somatic and sexual maturation, namely IGF-BP-1 and SBP [23]. A direct inhibiting effect of insulin has been demonstrated on the production of these two proteins by hepatoma cells in culture [30]. During puberty, insulin levels progressively rise, as a consequence of the physiological IR induced by the elevation of GH production [31]. IGF-BP-1 and SBP plasma levels decline throughout puberty, following a close inverse relationship with those of insulin [32]. Therefore, the physiological HI that accompanies puberty might be able to alter the bioactivity of sexual steroids and IGF-1 by influencing negatively their binding proteins. Interestingly, this action of insulin could be more efficient during the prepubertal and pubertal periods than in the adult life [30]. The negative effect of insulin on IGF-BP-1 production might have a great implication at the ovarian level since it could unbalance the intraovarian IGF systems [33], thereby leading to a greater intraovarian bioactivity of IGF-1 and/or IGF-2. In a provocative fashion, it could be proposed that the HI which accompanies (or induces?) PCOS does not interfere with ovarian insulin and/or IGF-1 receptors but acts merely through its hepatic effect on IGF binding proteins.

However so, the physiological effects of insulin during puberty could be exaggerated in those subjects who are genetically predisposed to IR and whose the HI could be worsened by the physiological IR of puberty. For the above-mentioned reasons, these subjects could be at risk to develop a PCOS at the time of adolescence. Although no clinical or experimental study directly supports this hypothesis, there are several indirect data which argue in favor [22]. First, PCOS often originates in puberty. Secondly, PCOS displays exaggerated features of puberty such as excessive cytochrome P-450 c17 activity in ovaries [34] as well as in adrenals [34, 35]. Thirdly, the gonadotropin secretion pattern in PCOS mimics and seems to amplify that of puberty [36]. Interestingly, it has been recently proposed that IGF-1 can produce an increase of GnRH release [37]. Lastly, IGF-BP-1 plasma levels are lower than normal in women with PCOS [38] and negatively correlated with plasma insulin levels [32]. Therefore, if one refers to the chronological events of puberty, it may be speculated that IR first induces an exaggerated adrenarche because of the loss of insulin inhibition of some adrenal enzyme functions [39]. Then, an exaggerated ovarian maturation would occur, with hyperactivity of the theca-interstitial compartment and subsequent inhibition of the granulosa cells. This could be due to the amplifying effect of HI on the intraovarian IGF system, which would favor the LH effects on theca-interstitial cells rather than the FSH action on granulosa cells. The pituitary secretion pattern of gonadotropins worsens this unbalance, since LH secretion is enhanced by the pulsatile pattern of GnRH secretion and the retroaction of estrogens arising from the aromatization of adrenal and ovarian androgens, while FSH secretion is either unaffected or impaired. Furthermore, an effect of HI on the hypothalamic pituitary system may also be evoked during puberty, via the activation of the local IGF systems [37].

Once the vicious circle is set up, it is conceivable that the insulin influence will decline over the years following puberty, once the physiological IR of puberty resorbs, leaving therefore the main role to gonadotropins. This hypothesis could explain the difficulties to obviate a direct relationship between insulin and androgens in adult women with common forms of PCOS and mild HI. On the other hand, this relation could 'reappear' in the rare observations of severe PCOS and high insulin plasma levels.

Conclusion

The insulin/IGF-1 hypothesis explaining the associations between HI and PCOS still needs strong support from clinical and experimental studies. It is our belief that if it turns out to be true, its main involvement should be during the pubertal period, with an exaggerated stimulation of the local (i.e. ovarian, adrenal, hypothalamic, pituitary) IGF systems [23]. Therefore, PCOS could still be considered as the consequence of a 'hyperpuberty', as has been suggested for many years [39]. The present hypothesis is less restrictive than the previous ones in that it involves not only the hypothalamic pituitary system, but the whole set of organs (i.e. ovaries, adrenals, pituitary, hypothalamus and liver) which interfere with the very complex phenomena of growth and puberty. Furthermore, the likely genetic origin of IR which accompanies some cases of PCOS could explain, at least in part, the genetic predisposition to this disease [40].

Acknowledgement

Thanks to Dr. J. Carew for kindly reviewing the English translation.

References

1 Dewailly D, Cortet-Rudelli C, Henric B, Longelin C, Fossati P: Insulinorésistance et syndrome des ovaires polymicrocystiques. Ann Endocrinol (Paris) 1992;53:1–7.

2 Kahn CR, Flier JS, Bar RS, Archer JA, Gorden P, Martin MM, Roth J: The syndromes of insulin resistance and acanthosis nigricans. Insulin-receptor disorders in man. N Engl J Med 1976; 294:739–745.

3 Dunaif A, Green G, Futterweit W, Dobrjanski A: Suppression of hyperandrogenism does not improve peripheral or hepatic insulin resistance in the polycystic ovary syndrome. J Clin Endocrinol Metab 1990;70:699–704.

4 Geffner ME, Kaplan SA, Bersch N, Golde DW, Landaw EM, Chang RJ: Persistence of insulin resistance in polycystic ovarian disease after inhibition of ovarian steroid secretion. Fertil Steril 1986;45:327–333.

5 Taylor SI, Kadowaki T, Kadowaki H, Accilli D, Cama A, Mc Keon C: Mutations in insulin receptor gene in insulin-resistant patients. Diabetes Care 1990;13:257–264.

6 Yamamoto R, Shiba T, Tobe K, Shibasaki Y, Koshio O, Izumi T, Odawara M, Mikami Y, Matsoora N, Akanuma Y, Takaku F, Kasuga M: Defect in tyrosine kinase activity of the insulin receptor from a patient with insulin resistance and acanthosis nigricans. J Clin Endocrinol Metab 1990;70:869–876.

7 Corenblum B, Baylis BW: Medical therapy for the syndrome of familial virilization, insulin resistance, and acanthosis nigricans. Fertil Steril 1990;53:421–425.

8 Burghen GA, Givens JR, Kitabchi AE: Correlation of hyperandrogenism with hyperinsulinism in polycystic ovarian disease. J Clin Endocrinol Metab 1980;50:113–116.

9 Shoupe CA, Kumar DD, Lobo RA: Insulin resistance in polycystic ovary syndrome. Am J Obstet Gynecol 1983;147:588–592.

10 Stuart CA, Peters EJ, Prince MJ, Richards G, Cavallo A, Meyer WJ: Insulin resistance with acanthosis nigricans: The roles of obesity and androgen excess. Metabolism 1986;35:197–205.

11 Smith S, Ravnikar VA, Barbieri RL: Androgen and insulin response to an oral glucose challenge in hyperandrogenic women. Fertil Steril 1987;48:72–77.

12 Conway GS, Jacobs HS, Holly JMP, Wass JAH: Effects of luteinizing hormone, insulin, insulin-like growth factor-I, and insulin-like growth factor small binding protein 1 in the polycystic ovary syndrome. Clin Endocrinol 1990;33:593–603.

13 Falcone T, Finegood DT, Fantus G, Morris D: Androgen response to endogenous insulin secretion during the frequently sampled intravenous glucose tolerance test in normal and hyperandrogenic women. J Clin Endocrinol Metab 1990;71:1653–1657.

14 Cortet-Rudelli C, Keuller H, Henric B, Longelin C, Fossati P, Dewailly D: Correlation between insulin plasma levels and clinical and biological features of polycystic ovarian disease. Clin Exp Endocrinol 1992 (in press).

15 Sharp PS, Kiddy DS, Reed MJ, Anyaoku V, Johnston DG, Franks S: Correlation of plasma insulin and insulin-like growth factor-I with indices of androgen transport and metabolism in women with polycystic ovary syndrome. Clin Endocrinol 1991;35:253–257.

16 Toscano V, Bianchi P, Balducci R, Guglielmi R, Mangiatini A, Lubrano C, Sciarra F: Lack of linear relationship between hyperinsulinaemia and hyperandrogenism. Clin Endocrinol 1992; 36:197–202.

17 Nestler JE, Barlascini CO, Matt DW, Steingold KA, Plymate SR, Clore JN, Blackard WG: Suppression of serum insulin by diazoxide reduces serum testosterone levels in obese women with polycystic ovary syndrome. J Clin Endocrinol Metab 1989;68:1027–1032.

18 Kiddy DS, Hamilton-Fairley D, Bush A, Short F, Anyaoku V, Reed MJ, Franks S: Improvement in endocrine and ovarian function during dietary treatment of obese women with polycystic ovary syndrome. Clin Endocrinol 1992; 36:105–111.

19 Poretsky L: On the paradox of insulin-induced hyperandrogenism in insulin-resistant states. Endocr Rev 1991;12:3–13.

20 Adashi EY, Resnick CE, D'Ercole AJ, Svoboda ME, Van Wyk JJ: Insulin-like growth factors as intraovarian regulators of granulosa cell growth and function. Endocr Rev 1985;6:400–420.

21 Barbieri RL, Makris A, Ryan KJ: Insulin stimulates androgen accumulation in incubations of human ovarian stroma and theca. Obstet Gynecol 1984;64:735–741.

22 Poretsky L, Kalin MF: The gonadotropic function of insulin. Endocr Rev 1987;8:132–141.

23 Nobels F, Dewailly D: Puberty and polycystic ovary syndrome: The insulin/insulin-like growth factor 1 (IGF-1) hypothesis. Fertil Steril 1992;58:655–666.

24 Levy MJ, Hernandez ER, Adashi EY, Stillman RJ, Roberts CT, LeRoith D: Expression of insulin-like growth factor (IGF)-I and II receptor genes during postnatal development of the rat ovary. 47th Annual Meeting of the American Fertility Society, Program Supplement. Fertil Steril 1991;S33.

25 Hillier SG, Yong EL, Illingworth PJ, Baird DT, Schwall RH: Effect of recombinant activin on androgen synthesis in cultured human thecal cells. J Clin Endocrinol Metab 1991;72:1206–1211.

26 Cara JF, Rosenfield RL: Insulin-like growth factor I and insulin potentiate luteinizing hormone-induced androgen synthesis by rat ovarian thecal-interstitial cells. Endocrinology 1988;123:733–739.

27 Penhoat A, Jaillard C, Saez JM: Synergistic effects of corticotropin and insulin-like growth factor I on corticotropin receptors and corticotropin responsiveness in cultured bovine adrenocortical cells. Biochem Biophys Res Commun 1989;165:355–359.

28 Dickerman Z, Grant DR, Faiman C, Winter JSD: Intraadrenal steroid concentrations in man: Zonal differences and developmental changes. J Clin Endocrinol Metab 1984;59:1031–1039.

29 Nestler JE, Strauss JF: Insulin as an effector of human ovarian and adrenal steroid metabolism. Clin Endocrinol Metab 1991;20:807–823.

30 Singh A, Hamilton-Fairley D, Koistinen R, Seppälä M, James VH, Franks S, Reed MJ: Effects of insulin-like growth factor-type I (IGF-I) and insulin on the secretion of sex hormone binding globulin and IGF-I binding protein (IBP-I) by human hepatoma cells. J Endocrinol 1990;124:R1.

31 Amiel SA, Caprio S, Sherwin RS, Plewe G, Haymond MW, Tamborlane WV: Insulin resistance of puberty: A defect restricted to peripheral glucose metabolism. J Clin Endocrinol Metab 1991;72:277–282.

32 Holly JMP, Smith CP, Dunger DB, Edge JA, Biddlecombe RA, Williams AJK, Howell R, Chard T, Savage MO, Rees LH, Wass JAH: Levels of the small insulin-like growth factor-binding protein are strongly related to those of insulin in prepubertal and pubertal children but only weakly so after puberty. J Endocrinol 1989;121:383–387.

33 Adashi EY, Resnick CE, Hurwitz A, Ricciarellie E, Hernandez ER, Roberts CT, Leroith D, Rosenfeld R: The intra-ovarian IGF system. Growth Regul 1991;2:10–15.

34 Rosenfield RL, Barnes RB, Cara JF, Lucky AW: Dysregulation of cytochrome P-450 c17 as the cause of polycystic ovarian syndrome. Fertil Steril 1990;53:785–791.

35 Dewailly D, Vantyghem M-C, Lemaire C, Dufosse F, Racadot A, Fossati P: Screening heterozygotes for 21-hydroxylase deficiency among hirsute women: Lack of utility of the adrenocorticotropin hormone test. Fertil Steril 1988;50:228–232.

36 Zumoff B, Freeman R, Compey S, Saenger P, Markowitz M, Kream J: A chronobiologic abnormality in luteinizing hormone secretion in teenage girls with the polycystic ovary syndrome. N Engl J Med 1983;309:1206–1211.

37 Hiney JK, Ojeda SR, Dees WL: Insulin-like growth factor I: A possible metabolic signal involved in the regulation of female puberty. Neuroendocrinology 1991;54:420–423.

38 Pekonen F, Laatikainen T, Buyalos R, Rutanen EM: Decreased 34 K insulin-like growth factor binding protein in polycystic ovarian disease. Fertil Steril 1989;51:972–975.

39 Yen SSC: Chronic anovulation caused by peripheral endocrine disorders; in Yen SSC, Jaffe RB (eds): Reproductive Endocrinology. Philadelphia, Saunders, 1991, pp 576–630.

40 Hague WM, Adams J, Reeders ST, Peto TEA, Jacobs HS: Familial polycystic ovaries: A genetic disease? Clin Endocrinol 1988;29:593–605.

Horm Res 1992;38:46–50

Charles Couet[a]
Jacques Delarue[a]
Thierry Constans[b]
Fernand Lamisse[a]

[a] Laboratoire de Nutrition et Clinique Médicale A, Hôpital Bretonneau, et
[b] Service de Gériatrie, Hôpital de l'Ermitage, Centre Hospitalier et Universitaire, Tours, France

Age-Related Insulin Resistance: A Review

Key Words
Aging
Insulin
Glucose
Metabolism

Abstract
Impaired glucose tolerance occurs with age. This impairment is multifactorial including a decrease in insulin-mediated glucose uptake by peripheral tissues and a delay in insulin-induced suppression of hepatic glucose output. A post-binding defect in insulin action such as a reduced capacity to transcribe more glucose transporter mRNA and/or a reduced translocation of preformed glucose transporters to plasma membrane is incriminated. However, insulin resistance with age is not a constant finding and other mechanism(s) has (have) to be involved in old individuals with impaired glucose tolerance and normal tissue insulin sensitivity.

Since the initial recognition by Spence [1], the impairment of oral and intravenous glucose tolerance with advancing age has been confirmed in the human [2, 3]. The assessment of the underlying mechanisms has led to discrepant conclusions probably because of the multifactorial process involved in the regulation of glucose homeostasis as well as the interference with confounding events associated with aging such as occult disease state, drug consumption, undernutrition, limited physical activity, changes in body composition, and reduced carbohydrate intake.

Although a decrease in noninsulin-mediated glucose disposal [4, 5] and a relative decline in β-cell responsiveness to a glucose challenge or a mixed meal [6] might contribute to the age-related glucose intolerance in man, it is the reduction of insulin action on target tissues which has received the bulk of attention. Therefore, this review will focus on the role of decreased insulin action in the deterioration of glucose tolerance in the elderly.

The combination of raised blood glucose levels and normal or even increased serum insulin concentrations in response to a glucose challenge has led to the concept that a decrease in insulin action, i.e., insulin resistance, is the main mechanism responsible for the age-related decline in glucose tolerance [2]. Since insulin is known to smooth down postprandial blood glucose concentrations by increasing the rate of glucose uptake by peripheral tissues (mainly the muscle tissue) and by decreasing the rate of hepatic glucose output, the question arises as to whether decreased insulin sensitivity takes place in peripheral tissue, in the liver, or both.

Peripheral Tissue Insulin Sensitivity

The effect of insulin on peripheral glucose uptake has been examined by several groups with different technical approaches. Using the euglycemic-hyperinsulinemic glu-

Charles Couet
Laboratoire de Nutrition et Clinique Médicale A
Hôpital Bretonneau
Centre Hospitalier et Universitaire
F–37044 Tours Cedex (France)

0301–0163/92/0382–0046
$2.75/0

cose clamp, a 28–54% decrease in the amount of glucose necessary to maintain euglycemia in the presence of similar serum insulin levels (~100 μU/ml) has been demonstrated in aged as compared to the young subjects [7–12]. Correction for the difference in lean body mass between young and old do not alter the conclusion [8, 10, 12]. Where examined, the dose-response relation between insulin concentrations and glucose infusion rates was shifted to the right in older individuals as compared to young adults [8, 10, 12]. There was however disagreement as to whether the maximal insulin response was also reduced with aging [8, 10, 12]. It is worth stressing that the variation in the insulin action observed in vivo between individuals was much greater among the older subjects [8, 9, 11]. For instance, Rosenthal et al. [9] reported that the coefficient of variation for glucose metabolic clearance measured during an euglycemic-hyperinsulinic clamp was doubled in the older (45%) compared with the young (23%) group. Similar observation can be made from other studies [8, 11] and indicates that a decrease in peripheral insulin sensitivity is not shared by all older subjects despite evidence of impaired glucose tolerance. Indeed, in two recent studies, Broughton et al. [13, 14] reported normal insulin sensitivity of peripheral tissue in highly selected groups of healthy elderly male subjects with impaired oral glucose tolerance test.

The assessment of insulin-stimulated glucose uptake across a muscle bed has confirmed the progressive loss of peripheral insulin sensitivity as a contributing factor for carbohydrate intolerance with age. In the presence of similar glucose and insulin levels, forearm glucose uptake in the elderly was found to be only one-third that of younger subjects [15]. Such conclusion was sustained by the results of a further expanded study performed by the same group [16]. Using this procedure, Kalant et al. [17] did not show an age-related decrease in insulin ability to promote peripheral glucose disposal but only 5 of the 31 subjects studied were over 49 years and only 1 subject was over the age of 60. In these studies, the rate of glucose uptake was normalized to forearm volume as an indicator of muscle mass. Whether the proportion of muscle and fat in the forearm vary with age remains to be clarified.

Finally, using a mathematical analysis of glucose and insulin curves obtained from the frequently sampled intravenous glucose tolerance test, Chen et al. [18] have found a 63% decrease in the insulin sensitivity index in the older subjects. The same group has demonstrated a significant improvement in both insulin release and insulin sensitivity when dietary carbohydrate intake of older individuals are increased from 45 to 85% of total calories. Such a dietary manipulation results in a net enhancement of glucose tolerance in response to both intravenous [19] and oral [20] glucose administration. This finding is consistent with the fact that populations eating spontaneous high carbohydrate diets exhibit no or less age-related insulin resistance [21].

Hepatic Insulin Sensitivity

Basal hepatic glucose output (HGO) was found to be unaffected by aging in all in vivo studies [4, 5, 7, 8, 11, 12, 14, 16] but one [22]. The ability of insulin to down-regulate HGO has been studied using the isotope dilution technique in association with the hyperinsulinic-euglycemic clamp by several authors. At low insulin infusion rate (15 $mU \cdot m^2 \cdot min^{-1}$), Fink et al. [8] observed that HGO was less suppressed in the elderly group (77 vs. 89%, old vs. young) despite higher serum insulin levels (61 vs. 33 $\mu U \cdot ml^{-1}$, old vs. young). In contrast, effective and even increased suppression of HGO has been reported in old individuals by Broughton et al. [14] for insulin concentration of 21 $\mu U \cdot ml^{-1}$. No age-related difference in the ability of insulin to reduce HGO is found when higher serum insulin levels are achieved (~90–120 $\mu U \cdot ml^{-1}$) [7, 8, 11]. Jackson et al. [16] have examined the turnover of glucose in the dynamic situation of an oral glucose tolerance test. They found that inhibition of HGO was delayed in onset but more prolonged in the elderly. The net result was a similar hepatic glucose conservation in elderly and control groups within the 270 min following an oral glucose load of 100 g. In this study, the delayed fall in HGO was associated with delayed insulin secretion.

Altogether, these data indicate that a decrease in peripheral tissue insulin sensitivity rather than in hepatic insulin sensitivity can be invoked as a contributing mechanism responsible for the age-related deterioration in carbohydrate tolerance. Nevertheless, other mechanism(s) must be involved wherever both impaired glucose tolerance and normal insulin sensitivity coexist in old individuals.

Possible Mechanisms beyond Insulin Resistance

The age-related insulin resistance observed in vivo indicates a defective insulin activity at the receptor and/or the postreceptor levels.

The right shift of the dose-response relation between insulin concentrations and rates of glucose uptake is a predicted consequence of a reduced number of receptors in a system in which spare receptors exist. Although decreased insulin receptor binding with age has been observed in human adipocytes [23, 24], most workers have reported normal insulin binding to human monocytes [10, 15], human and rat adipocytes [8, 25], cultured human fibroblasts [26] and stimulated lymphocytes [27]. Such data suggest that the decrease in insulin binding to its specific receptor is not the overriding defect beyond the age-related decrease in insulin sensitivity of peripheral tissues in vivo.

Alternatively, a diminished insulin sensitivity can be a consequence of a postbinding defect in insulin action. Increased glucose transport in muscle and fat tissues is one major cellular response to the insulin message following the formation of the insulin receptor complex. In these tissues, the insulin increases glucose transport by both a translocation of mainly one specific isoform of glucose transporters (GLUT4) from the intracellular low-density microsome pool to the plasma membrane [for reviews, see 28, 29] and an enhancement of the intrinsic activity of glucose transporters [30]. Using isolated human adipocytes, Fink et al. [31] have reported a 34% decrease in the maximum velocity (V_{max}) of insulin-stimulated 3-O-methylglucose transport in the elderly without any alteration in the affinity (K_m) of the transporter units. This finding is consistent with both a reduction in the number of glucose transporters with aging and a normal function of each transporter unit.

With respect to adipose tissue, it is conceivable that aging results in a depletion of total number of glucose transporters in keeping with the reduction in the amount of GLUT4 found in each subcellular fraction of adipose cell from aged obese rat [32, 33]. Adipose cellular enlargement goes with increased adiposity and aging in both the human [34–36] and the rat [32, 33]. Such enlargement of adipose cells is associated with insulin resistance and a relative depletion of glucose transport systems in the intracellular pool of large adipose cells is already known [32, 33]. In view of the minor role played by adipose tissue in the overall glucose utilization, it would be of limited interest to discuss further the relative importance of adipose cellular enlargement and aging per se in the age-related decline in glucose tolerance. Indeed, even though exercise elicits a protective action against the development of cell enlargement and adipocyte insulin resistance [37], it is primarily through an effect on the skeletal muscle and the liver [38] that physical training is likely to improve insulin-mediated glucose disposal in the elderly [39]. Insulin regulates the expression of GLUT4 isoform at the pretranslational level and both GLUT4 mRNA and GLUT4 isoform protein are increased by insulin in adipose cells [28, 29]. Whether aging results in a reduced capacity to transcribe more glucose transporter mRNA in response to insulin as it does for albumin mRNA in response to low protein intake [40] or hypoalbuminemia [41] remains to be established.

Although muscle tissue is the quantitatively most important tissue with respect to insulin-dependent glucose disposal, much less is known about the biological mechanism responsible for the insulin-stimulated glucose transport. Experimental difficulties associated with membrane isolation from muscle may account for this gap [29]. Therefore, it is uncertain whether reduction in total number of glucose transporters and/or decrease in their insulin-stimulated recruitment and translocation is the primary defect associated with the decline in insulin sensitivity of muscle tissue from aged humans. Despite the similarities reported between the hormonal regulation of glucose transporters in muscle and adipose tissue [29], there are both transporter and tissue specificities involved in the regulation of these proteins by insulin [28].

The site of the defect in the signaling pathway used by insulin to promote the translocation and the synthesis of intracellular glucose transporters might also differ according to the target tissue considering. For instance, normal insulin receptor tyrosine kinase activity was found in the liver of aged rats [42] whereas a modification with age was reported in rat adipocytes [43]. An age-related defect in the in vivo activation of the hepatic insulin receptor kinase resulting in reduced phosphorylation of its putative substrate pp180 have been recently documented [44]. A defect in recycling of the intracellular insulin receptor complex was demonstrated in adipocytes from older rats [45]. On the basis of the relationship observed between glucose transport and the processing of the intracellular insulin receptor complex, Trischitta and Reaven [45] suggested that the age-related abnormality of this processing might impede the insulin-stimulated translocation of glucose transport units to the plasma membrane as well as the recycling of receptor back to the cell membrane. In all likelihood, this mechanism does not appear of primary importance with respect to the insulin action on amino acid metabolism. Indeed, the reduced amino acid transport elicited in different cell types by drugs known to inhibit the intracellular processing of the insulin receptor complex [46] contrasts with the normal in vivo insulin sensitivity for amino acid disposal in the elderly [12, 47].

Studies on the intracellular metabolic fate of glucose indicate that transport was rate-limiting for glucose utilization [48, 49] and a decrease with age in the activity of several enzymes involved in glucose metabolism (hexokinase, phosphofructokinase, glycogen synthase and phosphorylase) has been found in either human adipocytes, rat muscle or rat liver [49–51]. Chanez et al. [52] have demonstrated that the time-related changes in the activity of numerous liver key enzymes involved in glycolysis and gluconeogenesis to starvation and to transition from high carbohydrate to high protein diet was delayed in the aged rat. The delay in the time-related changes in enzyme activities and in insulin/glucagon ratio were consistent. Such an age-related effect may contribute to reduce the adaptability to different dietary conditions.

According to the glucose-fatty acid cycle described by Randle et al. [53], the increased concentrations of plasma free fatty acids (FFA) wigh aging found in most [2, 15] but not all studies [54] might antagonize the insulin-stimulated glucose transport activity [55, 56]. As recently reviewed by Jackson [57], several but indirect findings argue against a causative effect of increased fasting plasma FFA levels in the age-related carbohydrate intolerance. However, the role played by high FFA concentrations in the reduction of insulin sensitivity in aged humans requires to be addressed more specifically in further studies before a final conclusion can be made. Indeed, raised plasma FFA levels, elevated rate of lipid oxidation and decreased rate of glucose oxidation have been documented in aged compared to young individuals after both glucose and fructose ingestion [58]. Since fructose bypasses the defect in insulin-stimulated glucose transport, the reduced increment in carbohydrate oxidation seen after fructose ingestion in the old as compared to the young suggests that a defect distal to the transport glucose system is also involved in the age-related insulin resistance.

In conclusion, a decreased insulin sensitivity can contribute to the age-related carbohydrate intolerance. The impairment of insulin action is mainly exhibited in peripheral tissues and is due to a postreceptor defect. A reduced capacity to transcribe more glucose transporter mRNA in response to insulin stimulation and a decreased ability of insulin to induce translocation of preformed glucose transporters to the plasma membrane could be involved in this defect. However, other mechanism(s) has (have) to take place in old individuals with impaired glucose tolerance and normal tissue insulin sensitivity. Finally, considerable effort must be put in controlling for confounding variables known to worsen glucose homeostasis in a synergistic fashion.

References

1 Spence JW: Some observations on sugar tolerance with special reference to variation found at different ages. Q J Med 1921;14:314–326.
2 Davidson MB: The effect of ageing on carbohydrate metabolism: A review of the English literature and a practical approach to the diagnosis of diabetes mellitus in the elderly. Metabolism 1979;28:688–705.
3 De Fronzo RA: Glucose intolerance and aging. Diabetes Care 1981;4:493–501.
4 Meneilly GS, Elahi D, Minaker KL, et al: Impairment of noninsulin-mediated glucose disposal in the elderly. J Clin Endocrinol Metab 1989;68:566–571.
5 Paolisso G, Marrazzo G, De Riu S, et al: Effects of mild-to-moderate hyperglycemia per se on glucose production and uptake in the elderly. Eur J Med 1992;1:6–12.
6 Gumbiner B, Polonsky KS, Beltz WF, et al: Effects of aging on insulin secretion. Diabetes 1989;38:1549–1556.
7 De Fronzo RA: Glucose intolerance and aging. Evidence for tissue insensitivity to insulin. Diabetes 1979;28:1095–1101.
8 Fink RI, Kolterman OG, Griffin J, et al: Mechanisms of insulin resistance in aging. J Clin Invest 1983;71:1523–1535.
9 Rosenthal M, Doberne L, Greenfield M, et al: Effect of age on glucose tolerance, insulin secretion and in vivo insulin action. J Am Geriatr Soc 1982;30:562 567.
10 Rowe JW, Minaker KL, Pallotta JA: Characterization of the insulin resistance of aging. J Clin Invest 1983;71:1581–1587.
11 Pagano G, Cassader M, Cavallo-Perin P, et al: Insulin resistance in the aged: A quantitative evaluation of in vivo insulin sensitivity and in vitro glucose transport. Metabolism 1984;33: 976–981.
12 Fukagawa NK, Minaker KL, Rowe JW, et al: Glucose and amino acid metabolism in aging man: Differential effects of insulin. Metabolism 1988;37:371–377.
13 Broughton DL, Alberti KG, James OF, et al: Peripheral tissue insulin sensitivity in healthy elderly subjects. Gerontology 1987;33:357–362.
14 Broughton DL, James OW, Alberti KG, et al: Peripheral and hepatic insulin sensitivity in healthy elderly human subjects. Eur J Clin Invest 1991;21:13–21.
15 Jackson RA, Blix PM, Matthews JA, et al: Influence of ageing on glucose homeostasis. J Clin Endocrinol Metab 1982;55:840–848.
16 Jackson RA, Hawa MI, Roshania RD, et al: Influence of aging on hepatic and peripheral glucose metabolism in humans. Diabetes 1988; 37.119–129.
17 Kalant N, Leibovici D, Leibovici T, et al: Effect of age on glucose utilization and responsiveness to insulin in forearm muscle. J Am Geriatr Soc 1980;28:304–307.
18 Chen M, Bergman RN, Pacini G, et al: Pathogenesis of age-related glucose intolerance in man: Insulin resistance and decreased B-cell function. J Clin Endocrinol Metab 1985;60: 13–20.
19 Chen M, Bergman RN, Porte D Jr: Insulin resistance and B-cell dysfunction in aging: The importance of dietary carbohydrate. J Clin Endocrinol Metab 1988;67:951–957.
20 Chen M, Halter JB, Porte D Jr: The role of dietary carbohydrate in the decreased glucose tolerance in the elderly. J Am Geriatr Soc 1987; 35:417–424.
21 Pacini G, Valerio A, Beccaro F, et al: Insulin sensitivity and beta-cell responsivity are not decreased in elderly subjects with normal OGTT. J Am Geriatr Soc 1988;36:317–323.

22 Robert JJ, Cummins JC, Wolfe RR, et al: Quantitative aspects of glucose production and metabolism in healthy elderly subjects. Diabetes 1982;31:203–211.
23 Pagano G, Cassader M, Diana A, et al: Insulin resistance in the aged: The role of the peripheral insulin receptors. Metabolism 1981;30: 46–49.
24 Bolinder J, Östman J, Arner P: Influence of aging on insulin receptor binding and metabolic effects of insulin on human adipose tissue. Diabetes 1983;32:959–964.
25 Olefsky JM, Reaven GM: Effects of age and obesity on insulin binding to isolated adipocytes. Endocrinology 1975;96:1486–1498.
26 Hollenberg ND, Schneider EL: Receptor for insulin and epidermal growth factor-urogastrone in adult human fibroblasts do not change with donor age. Mech Ageing Dev 1979;11:37–43.
27 Helderman JH: Constancy of pharmacokinetic properties of the lymphocyte insulin receptor during aging. J Gerontol 1980;35:329–334.
28 Kahn BB, Flier JS: Regulation of glucose transporter gene expression in vitro and in vivo. Diabetes Care 1990;13:548–564.
29 Kasanicki MA, Pilch PF: Regulation of glucose transporter function. Diabetes Care 1990;13: 219–227.
30 Kahn BB, Shulman GI, DeFronzo RA, et al: Normalization of blood glucose in diabetic rats with phlorizin treatment reverses insulin-resistant glucose transport in adipose cells without restoring glucose transporter gene expression. J Clin Invest 1991;87:561–570.
31 Fink RI, Wallace P, Olefsky JM: Effects of aging on glucose-mediated glucose disposal and glucose transport. J Clin Invest 1986;77:2034–2041.
32 Hissin PJ, Foley JE, Wardzala LJ, et al: Mechanism of insulin-resistant glucose transport activity in the enlarged adipose cell of the aged, obese rat. J Clin Invest 1982;70:780–790.
33 Ezaki O, Fukuda N, Itakura H: Role of two types of glucose transporters in enlarged adipocytes from aged obese rats. Diabetes 1990;39: 1543–1549.
34 Cohn SH, Vartsky D, Yasumura S, et al: Compartmental body composition based on total-body nitrogen, potassium and calcium. Am J Physiol 1980;239:E524–E530.
35 Borkan G, Hults DE, Gerzof SG, et al: Age changes in body composition revealed by computed tomography. J Gerontol 1983;38:673–677.
36 Björntorp P: Effects of age, sex and clinical conditions on adipose tissue cellularity in man. Metabolism 1974;23:1091–1102.
37 Craig BW, Garthwaite SM, Holloszy JO: Adipocyte insulin resistance: Effects of aging, obesity, and food restriction. J Appl Physiol 1987; 62:95–100.
38 Rodnick KJ, Haskell WL, Swislocki ALM, et al: Improved insulin action in muscle, liver and adipose tissue in physically trained human subjects. Am J Physiol 1987;253:E489–E495.
39 Hollenbeck CB, Haskell WL, Rosenthal M, et al: Effect of habitual physical exercice on regulation of insulin-stimulated glucose disposal in older males. J Am Geriatr Soc 1986;33:273–277.
40 Pain VM, Clemens MJ, Garlick PJ: The effect of protein deficiency on albumin synthesis and the concentration of active messenger ribonucleic acid in the rat liver. Biochem J 1978;172: 129–135.
41 Zähringer J, Baliga BS, Munro HN: Increased levels of microsomal albumin mRNA in the liver of nephrotic rats. FEBS Lett 1976;62: 322.
42 Bryer-Ash M, Freidenberg GR: The insulin resistance of aging resides at a site distal to the insulin receptor kinase in Fisher rat (abstract). Diabetes 1987(suppl 1):56A.
43 Andres A, Pulido JA; Satrustegui J, et al: The kinase activity of the insulin receptor is modified during ageing (abstract). Diabetologia 1987;30:494A.
44 Nadiv O, Cohen O, Zick Y: Defects in insulin's signal transduction in old rat livers. Endocrinology 1992;130:1515–1524.
45 Trischitta V, Reaven GM: Evidence of a defect in insulin receptor recycling in adipocytes from older rats. Am J Physiol 1988;254:E39–E44.
46 Peavy DE, Edmondson JW, Duckworth WC: Selective effects of inhibitors of hormone processing of insulin action in isolated hepatocytes. Endocrinology 1984;114:753–760.
47 Fukagawa NK, Minaker K, Young VR, et al: Leucine metabolism in aging humans: Effect of insulin and substrate availability. Am J Physiol 1989;256:E288–E294.
48 Fink RI, Kolterman OG, Kao M, et al: The role of the transport glucose system in the postreceptor defect in insulin action associated with human aging. J Clin Endocrinol Metab 1984; 58:721–725.
49 Goodman MN, Dluz SM, McElaney MA, et al: Glucose uptake and insulin sensitivity in rat muscle: Changes during 3–96 weeks of age. Am J Physiol 1983;244:E93–E100.
50 Belfiore F, Vagroni G, Napoli E, et al: Effects of ageing on key enzymes of glucose metabolism in human adipose tissue. J Mol Med 1977; 2:89–95.
51 Khandelwal RJ, Enno TL, Narayanan N: Effects of age on glycogen synthase and phosphorylase activities in rat liver. Mech Ageing Dev 1984;28:13–22.
52 Chanez M, Bois-Joyeux B, Peret J: Age-dependent changes in rat hepatic fructose 2,6-biphosphate, 6-phosphofructo-2-kinase/fructose 2,6-biphosphatase and pyruvate kinase activity in response to high protein diet or starvation. Diabete Metab 1988;14:80–87.
53 Randle PJ, Garland PB, Hales CN, et al: The glucose-fatty acid cycle: Its role in insulin sensitivity and the metabolic disturbances of diabetes mellitus. Lancet 1963;i:785–789.
54 Rosenthal MJ, Woodside WF: Nocturnal regulation of free fatty acids in healthy young and elderly men. Metabolism 1988;37:645–648.
55 Brady LJ, Goodman MN, Kalish FN, et al: Insulin binding and sensitivity in rat skeletal muscle: Effect of starvation. Am J Physiol 1981;240:E184–E190.
56 Simpson IA, Cushman SW: Hormonal regulation of mammalian glucose transport. Annu Rev Biochem 1986;55:1059–1089.
57 Jackson RA: Mechanisms of age-related glucose intolerance. Diabetes Care 1990;13(suppl 2):9–19.
58 Simonson DC, Tappy L, Jequier E, et al: Normalization of carbohydrate-induced thermogenesis by fructose in insulin-resistant states. Am J Physiol 1988;245:E201–E207.

Horm Res 1992;38:51–56

B. Vialettes
P. Silvestre

Service de Médecine Interne et Nutrition, CHU La Timone, Marseille, France

Pharmacological Approach in the Treatment of Insulin Resistance

Key Words
Insulin
Biguanides
Sulfonylureas
Insulin resistance

Abstract
Insulin resistance syndromes are heterogeneous in either severity or mechanism. Many drugs have been shown to counteract various elements of insulin resistance. Some of them, by normalization of metabolic parameters, decrease insulin resistance induced by chronic hyperglycemia in diabetes. Insulin and, to some extent, sulfonylureas are in this group, but these drugs are not stricto sensu medication of insulin resistance. Some drugs sensitize peripheral tissues to the action of insulin. For instance, biguanides and thiazolidine-dione facilitate translocation to the membrane of glucose transporter in presence of insulin. Other compounds as vanadate or IGF-1 mimic some peripheral action of insulin. Finally, blockade of FFA oxidation by specific inhibitors (methylpalmoxyrate) can limit insulin resistance. In 1992, among these compounds, specific of insulin resistance, biguanides are mostly used. However, the efficacy of these drugs is moderate and limited to type 2 diabetes.

Insulin resistance is likely to be the first mechanism which leads to type 2 diabetes. It is associated with numerous other risk factors of atherosclerosis in the context of syndrome X. It would therefore be of enormous benefit to discover an efficient drug which specifically acts on insulin resistance. Unfortunately, insulin resistance is polymorphic. The severe insulin resistance syndromes in which enormous amounts of insulin are unable to overcome, are quite different from insulin resistance associated with type 2 diabetes. There are several examples of dissociation of insulin sensitivity in the triad of liver, muscle and adipose tissue. In addition, even at the cellular level, receptor and postreceptor defects have been described. In addition, we must keep in mind that chronic hyperglycemia can also generate 'secondary metabolic insulin resistance', adding to the initial disorder. All these reasons explain why we do not have an ideal therapeutic agent effective against insulin resistance at our disposal. It is also difficult to know precisely the mechanism of the action of existing drugs.

The aim of this review is to analyze the efficacy of the drugs which are currently available and give information on the compounds which potentially could be of benefit in the treatment of insulin resistance states in the future.

Dr. B. Vialettes
Service de Médecine Interne et Nutrition
CHU La Timone
bd Jean-Moulin
F–13385 Marseille Cedex 5 (France)

0301–0163/92/0382–0051
$2.75/0

Treatment of 'Secondary Metabolic Insulin Resistance' by Insulin

Chronic hyperglycemia itself can induce peripheral insulin resistance by reducing the number of glucose transporters in insulin-sensitive tissues [reviewed in 1]. In both uncontrolled type 1 and type 2 diabetes, this secondary metabolic resistance may worsen the disorder. Therefore, intensified insulin therapy directed at normalizing plasma glucose could be useful. In type 1 diabetes, a beneficial effect of intensified insulin pump therapy has been reported by Yki-Jarvinen and Koivisto [2]. After 6 weeks of pump treatment every patient, with the exception of 1, exhibited an improvement in the glucose metabolic clearance rate and a decrease of basal hepatic glucose production. In type 2 diabetes characterized by a specific form of insulin resistance, results are less convincing. Boden et al. [3] have shown that very modest glycemic improvement by dietary fiber supplementation, improved carbohydrate oxidation, but carbohydrate storage remained suppressed. In addition, Nankervis et al. [4] have shown that a conventional insulin treatment applied to uncontrolled type 2 diabetic patients suppressed basal hepatic glucose production but did not influence peripheral glucose uptake. Finally, Ginsberg and Rayfield [5] have treated 15 obese diabetic patients with insulin for 4–8 weeks. They noted a significant improvement of insulin sensitivity evaluated by the SSPG test in all patients. However, in this heterogenous group of subjects, insulin resistance totally disappeared after insulin therapy in only 5. We conclude that in type 2 diabetic patients who are severely insulin-resistant, glucose normalization induced by insulin only partially improves insulin sensitivity.

Recombinant proinsulin has been proposed as an insulin agonist particularly useful in the treatment of insulin resistance [6]. Recombinant proinsulin has greater effects in suppressing hepatic glucose production than in stimulating glucose disposal. Unfortunately, clinical studies were inconclusive as proinsulin induced severe hypoglycemia.

Oral Hypoglycemic Agents

Biguanides

Biguanides are compounds which have been used in the treatment of type 2 diabetes since the 1950s. Metformin is the most extensively used biguanide as it induces less lactic acidosis than others including, for example, fenformin. Properties of the biguanides combine a reduction in plasma glucose, and an improvement in lipid parameters in type 2 diabetic patients without the risk of hypoglycemia. They are efficient only in the presence of insulin and do not induce insulin secretion by β cells. They seem to act by increasing insulin sensitivity.

In type 1 diabetes several studies [reviewed in 7] have shown that metformin added to intensified insulin therapy leads to a significant decrease of glycemia and a 25–50% reduction of insulin needs, especially during mealtimes. In type 2 diabetic patients, metformin decreases plasma glucose without increasing plasma insulin. This effect is mainly mediated by the increase of peripheral glucose disposal according to Hother-Nielsen et al. [8] and by the suppression of basal hepatic glucose production according to Jackson et al. [9].

The precise mechanism of action is still poorly understood, and appears to be multifactorial. The biguanide effects on membrane expression of insulin receptors are still the object of debate. Some authors argue that biguanides induce an increase in receptor numbers on circulating blood cells in treated patients, or on cell lines following in vitro incubation with metformin [10–12]. However, these results have not been confirmed by other studies [13, 14]. More recently, tyrosine kinase activity of isolated receptors has been studied after in vitro incubation and in vivo treatment with metformin. Results are also divergent. Grigorescu et al. [15] have found that metformin increased tyrosine kinase activity of the insulin receptor of a particular cell, *Xenopus larvis* ovocyte. Rossetti et al. [16] have noted the same phenomenon on skeletal muscle cell isolated from metformin-treated rats. But, in contrast, Matthaei and Greten [17] did not find such an effect on rat adipocytes incubated in presence of metformin. These conflicting results show that metformin's effect on insulin receptors is variable and depends on cell types and experimental design. Therefore, we can conclude that the main location of the metabolic effect of metformin is at the postreceptor level [18]. Biguanides increase glucose uptake by muscle cells [19] and adipocytes [17]. This effect is mediated by a potentiation of glucose transporter translocation induced by insulin [17]. Finally, metformin is a potent suppressor of hepatic neoglycogenesis [20].

Several clinical studies in type 2 diabetics have also shown that biguanides are able to reduce other risk factors of atherosclerosis which are associated with insulin resistance in syndrome X. Metformin can decrease blood pressure [21], triglycerides [14, 21, 22] and abnormalities of fibrinolysis [reviewed in 23] in noninsulin-dependent diabetic patients. In conclusion, biguanides are the main group of drugs used worldwide, which have proven activity against the insulin resistance syndrome associated with type 2 diabetes. Unfortunately, this effect remains relatively modest as these drugs are rarely or not effective when treating severe insulin resistance syndromes with profound abnormalities of insulin binding or phosphorylation of receptors.

Sulfonylureas

The sulfonylureas are another class of oral antidiabetic agents which are largely used in the treatment of type 2 diabetes [24]. They are potent insulin secretagogues acting on ATP-sensitive potassium-ion channels of β cells. Their chief effect in vivo is to increase β cell sensitivity to glucose and adapt the insulin response to hyperglycemia. For the last 10 years, several extrapancreatic effects of these drugs have been described, but their relevance to the antidiabetic action of sulfonylureas remains controversial.

During chronic treatment of type 2 diabetic patients by sulfonylureas, plasma glucose decreases but surprisingly the parallel insulin increment is usually modest or even absent in some subjects. This finding suggests that these compounds might act on insulin sensitivity of peripheral tissues in addition to insulin release. Indeed, Greenfield et al. [25], Best et al. [26], Kolterman et al. [27], and Ward et al. [28] have demonstrated that noninsulin-dependent diabetics treated with sulfonylureas exhibited both an increase of glucose metabolic clearance rate and a suppression of basal hepatic glucose production. This peripheral effect occurred early at 3 months and could be even greater during long-term treatment. In two of these studies, responder patients were characterized by a better improvement of insulin sensitivity than stimulation of insulin secretion. However, it is very difficult in these studies to differentiate between a direct role of sulfonylureas on target tissues or an indirect effect mediated by the normalization of plasma glucose, particularly in responder patients.

In vitro experiments have demonstrated the extrapancreatic activity of sulfonylureas. The beneficial effect of these compounds on insulin receptor function of blood cells or insulin-dependent tissues, which has been previously suggested by Prince and Olefsky [24], has not been confirmed. Vigneri et al. [12] have studied four sulfonylureas (tolbutamide, glyburide, glycazide and glycosamide) on cell lines of four origins (lymphocyte, hepatocyte, fibroblast, epithelial cell). In every combination, none of the sulfonylureas used influenced the number or affinity of insulin receptors. Identical results have been reported by Salhanick et al. [30] on hepatocytes and Maloff and Lockwood [31] on adipocytes. More recently, Bak et al. [32] did not find any change in the insulin receptor on skeletal muscle cells taken from patients chronically treated with glycazide. These results suggest that extrapancreatic effects of sulfonylureas are likely to be localized at the postreceptor level. Sulfonylureas by either enhancement of insulin action or insulinomimetic action increase the uptake of glucose by muscle cells [32] or adipocytes [33]. Recent publications suggest that this cellular effect could be mediated by the enhancement of translocation of glucose transporters towards the external membrane of the cell [34, 35]. Finally, sulfonylureas could also stimulate activity of glycogen synthase as shown by Bak et al. [32] on cell culture and Nyomba et al. [36] on muscle biopsy.

However, despite this evidence, the potency of sulfonylureas in the treatment of insulin resistance remains doubtful. Indeed, in type 1 diabetes in which secondary insulin resistance has been documented, these hypoglycemic agents are unable to reduce insulin requirements evaluated by automatized insulin delivery devices, and even insulin resistance measured by glucose clamp studies [37–40]. Only two discordant voices reported a mild improvement in insulin sensitivity, and then at low insulin concentrations [41, 42]. Finally, in one case report [43] of a massive intoxication by glibenclamide in a diabetic patient rendered insulinopenic by partial pancreatectomy, no hypoglycemic attack occurred despite very high sulfonylurea blood levels. All these elements suggest that extrapancreatic effects of sulfonylureas, mimicking or enhancing insulin action, are of relatively low clinical relevance.

Potential Treatments of Insulin Resistance

Thiazolidine-Dione

These compounds which have some structural similarities with sulfonylureas and biguanides are insulin-enhancers. Some molecules have been tested in animal models, e.g. ciglitazone [44], CS-045 [45] and englitazone [46]. They have a hypoglycemic activity especially in animal models characterized by an insulin resistance as KK, ob/ob, db/db mice or Zucker rats. In contrast, ciglitazone has no effect in lean glucose-tolerant animals or in insulinopenic diabetic animals. These drugs seem to offer specific treatment for insulin resistance. The mechanism of action has been localized downstream to the insulin receptor. All the insulin-sensitive tissues are affected. In the liver, glyconeogenesis is suppressed and glucose incorporation into proteins and lipids enhanced. In the adipocyte, the oxidation and incorporation into lipids of carbohydrates is increased. Muscle uptake of glucose is also stimulated. Other effects such as repletion of insulin granules in β cells or increases of low affinity insulin binding sites on target cells are likely to be secondary to the decrease of hyperinsulinism.

In vitro, these molecules enhance the insulin-induced uptake of glucose. They can also abolish isoprenaline-induced insulin resistance [44]. The mechanism of action is an enhancement of insulin-induced translocation of the glucose transporter. In contrast, affinity of the transporter for glucose is not changed [44]. These substances which seem to be a specific treatment of insulin resistance have been recently tested in man. Suter et al. [47] have reported a pilot study using CS-045 in 11 obese noninsulin-dependent diabetics. Of the 11 patients, 8 exhibited a clinical response as manifested by lower fasting plasma glucose (−18% in the total group, −38% in the responders) after 3–10 weeks. This improvement in glycemic control was associated with decreases in plasma insulin, triglycerides and FFA concentrations. Basal hepatic glucose production was also suppressed and peripheral glucose disposal increased. These results are promising and suggest that these compounds could be potentially important in the treatment of insulin resistance in the future.

Vanadium [reviewed in 48, 49]

Vanadium salts (vanadate and vanadyle) can mimic insulin activity. In normal rats, administration of vanadium decreases plasma insulin levels without inducing hypoglycemia. In streptozotocin-induced diabetic rats, vanadium normalizes plasma glucose despite a persistent low level of insulin. All the peripheral metabolic activities of insulin could be reproduced with vanadium; stimulation of glycolysis and glyconeogenesis in the liver, inhibition of lipolysis and enhancement of liposynthesis in adipocyte, and an increase of hexose uptake and glycogen synthase activity in skeletal muscle cell. This metabolic effect has also been reported in animal models of diabetes characterized by major insulin resistance as fa/fa rats and ob/ob or db/db mice [50]. The mechanism of this activity is controversial. Vanadium could interfere with the insulin receptor activity, by either inhibiting dephosphorylation of tyrosine sites of the receptor by specific phosphatases or by itself inducing the autophosphorylation of tyrosine residues. It could also stimulate the translocation of glucose transporters GLUT-1 and GLUT-4 toward the cell membrane. Experimental results in animal models are encouraging for the future but the toxic risks [51] have to be taken into consideration.

FFA Oxidation Inhibitors

It is well known since Randle's work [52] that FFA oxidation is a factor which enhances hepatic glucose production and limits peripheral glucose uptake. Some substances such as methylpalmoxyrate can competitively inhibit long chain FFA oxidation in the liver. Methylpalmoxyrate administered to the streptozotocin-induced diabetic rat decreases plasma glucose and hepatic glycogenosynthesis [52]. This drug has been used in a case of severe insulin resistance in a patient with anti-insulin receptor autoantibodies [53]. In this patient a short-term treatment led to a 25% decrease of plasma glucose and a reduction of RQ (suggesting a better balance between carbohydrate and lipid oxidation). Hepatic glucose production and neoglycogenesis from lactate and alanine were also decreased.

Other Substances

Other compounds, in animal models, have shown potential activity against insulin resistance, for example hydroxypropionic acid which is an inhibitor of gluconeogenesis [54] and β-adrenergic agonists which decrease hepatic glucose production and increase muscular glucose oxidation [55, 56].

Recombinant human insulin-like growth factor 1 (rhIGF-1) has been evaluated in major insulin resistance syndromes in humans. The results have shown that rhIGF-1 minimized glycemia, plasma insulin and C-peptide levels, probably by acting through the type 1 IGF receptor in striated muscle and other tissues [57, 58].

In conclusion, the pharmacological treatment of insulin resistance in 1992 can be summarized by (1) obtaining good glycemic control, whatever the means (insulin or oral hypoglycemic agents), and (2) the use of biguanides which, among the oral hypoglycemic agents, have the greatest effect on insulin resistance. Unfortunately, the efficacy of this approach is relatively modest and the pharmacological treatment of insulin resistance has still to be discovered.

References

1 Yki-Jarvinen H: Acute and chronic effects of hyperglycaemia on glucose metabolism. Diabetologia 1990;33:579–585.
2 Yki-Jarvinen H, Koivisto VA: Continuous subcutaneous insulin infusion therapy decreases insulin resistance in type 1 diabetes. J Clin Endocrinol Metab 1984;58:659–666.
3 Boden G, Ray TK, Smith RH, Owen DE: Carbohydrate oxidation and storage in obese non-insulin-dependent diabetic patients; Effect of improving glycemic control. Diabetes 1983;32: 982–987.
4 Nankervis A, Proietto J, Aiken P, Harewood N, Alford F: Differential effects of insulin therapy on hepatic and peripheral insulin sensitivity in type 2 (non-insulin-dependent). Diabetologia 1982;23:320–325.
5 Ginsberg H, Rayfield EJ: Effect of insulin on insulin resistance in type 2 diabetic subjects: Evidence for heterogeneity. Diabetes 1981;30: 739–745.
6 Lebovitz HE: Newer non-sulfonylurea agents for the management of hyperglycaemia in patients with NIDDM; in Alberti KGMM, Krall LP (eds): The Diabetes Annual 4. Amsterdam, Elsevier, 1988, pp 67–79.
7 Slama G: The insulin-sparing effect of metformin in insulin-treated diabetic patients. Diabete Metab 1991;17:241–243.
8 Hother-Nielsen O, Schmitz O, Andersen PH, Beck-Nielsen H, Pedersen O: Metformin improves peripheral but not hepatic insulin action in obese patients with type 2 diabetes. Acta Endocrinol (Copenh) 1989;120:257–265.
9 Jackson RA, Hawa Mi, Jaspan JB, Sim BM, Disilvio L, Featherbe D, Kurtl AB: Mechanism of metformin action in non-insulin-dependent diabetes. Diabetes 1987;36:632–640.
10 Holle A, Mangels W, Dreyer M, Kuhnan J, Rudiger HW: Biguanide treatment increases the number of insulin receptor sites on human erythrocytes. N Engl J Med 1981:305:563–566.
11 Lord JM, White SI, Bailey CJ: Effect of metformin on insulin receptor binding and glycaemic control in type 2 diabetes. BMJ 1983;286:830–831.
12 Vigneri R, Pezzino V, Wong KY, Goldfine ID: Comparison of the in vitro effects of biguanides and sulfonylureas on insulin binding to the receptor in target cells. J Clin Endocrinol Metab 1982;54:95–100.
13 Prager R, Schernthaner G: Insulin receptor binding to monocytes, insulin secretion and glucose tolerance following metformin treatment. Results of a double-blind cross-over study in type 2 diabetics. Diabetes 1983;32: 1083–1086.
14 Wu MS, Johnston P, Sheu WHH, Hollenbeck CB, Jeng CY, Goldfine ID, Chen YDI, Reaven GM: Effect of metformin on carbohydrate and lipoprotein metabolism in NIDDM patients. Diabetes Care 1990;13:1–8.
15 Grigorescu F, Laurent A, Chavanieu A, Capony JP: Cellular mechanism of metformin action. Diabete Metab 1991;17:146–149.
16 Rossetti L, De Fronzo RA, Gherzi R, Stein P, Andraghetti G, et al: Effects of metformin treatment on insulin action in diabetic rats: In vitro correlation. Metabolism 1990;39:425–435.
17 Matthaei S, Greten H: Evidence that metformin ameliorates cellular insulin resistance by potentiating translocation of glucose transporters to the membrane. Diabete Metab 1991;17: 150–158.
18 Fantus IG, Brosseau R: Mechanism of action of metformin: Insulin receptor and post-receptor effects in vitro and in vivo. J Clin Endocrinol Metab 1986;63:898–905.
19 Galuska D, Zierath J, Thorne A, Sonnefeld T, Wallberg-Henriksson H: Metformin increases insulin stimulated glucose transport in insulin resistance human skeletal muscle. Diabete Metab 1991;17:159–163.
20 Meyer F, Ipakthi M, Clauser H: Specific inhibition of gluconeogenesis by biguanides. Nature 1967;213:203–204.
21 Landin K, Tengborn L, Smith U: Treating insulin resistance in hypertension with metformin reduces both blood pressure and metabolic risk factors. J Intern Med 1991;229:181–187.
22 Schneider J: Effects of metformin on dyslipoproteinemia in non-insulin-dependent diabetes mellitus. Diabete Metab 1991;17:185–190.
23 Grant PJ: The effects of metformin on the fibrinolytic systems in diabetic and non-diabetic subjects. Diabete Metab 1991;17:168–173.
24 Gerich JE: Oral hypoglycemic agents. N Engl J Med 1989;321: 1231–1245.
25 Greenfield MS, Doberne L, Rosenthal M, Schultz B, Widstrom A, Reaven GM: Effect of sulfonylurea treatment on in vivo insulin secretion and action in patients with non-insulin-dependent diabetes mellitus. Diabetes 1982; 31:307–312.
26 Best JD, Judzewitski G, Pfeifer MA, Beard JC, Halter JB, Porte D: The effect of chronic sulfonylurea therapy on hepatic glucose production in non-insulin-dependent diabetes. Diabetes 1982;31:333–338.
27 Kolterman OG, Gray RS, Shapiro G, Scarlett JA, Griffin J, Olefsky JM: The acute and chronic effects of sulfonylurea therapy in type 2 diabetic subjects. Diabetes 1984;33:346–354.
28 Ward G, Harrison LC, Proietto J, Aitken P, Nankervis A: Glyclazide therapy is associated with potentiation of postbinding insulin action in obese, non-insulin-dependent diabetic subjects. Diabetes 1985;34:241–245.
29 Prince MJ, Olefsky JM: Direct in vitro effect of a sulfonylurea to increase human fibroblast insulin receptors. J Clin Invest 1980;66:608–611.
30 Salhanick AI, Konowitz P, Amatruda JM: Potentiation of insulin action by a sulfonylurea in primary cultures of hepatocytes from normal and diabetic rats. Diabetes 1983;32:206–212.
31 Maloff BL, Lockwood DH: In vitro effects of a sulfonylurea on insulin action in adipocytes. Potentiation of insulin-stimulated hexose transport. J Clin Invest 1981;68:85.
32 Bak JF, Schmitz O, Sorensen NS, Pedersen O: Post-receptor effects of sulfonylurea on skeletal muscle glycogen synthase activity in type 2 diabetic patients. Diabetes 1989;38:1343–1350.
33 Davidson MB, Molnar G, Fuurman A, Yamagushi D: Glyburide-stimulated glucose transport in cultured muscle cells via protein C-mediated pathway requiring new protein synthesis. Diabetes 1991;40:1531–1538.
34 Wang PH, Moller D, Flier JS, Nayak RC, Smith RJ: Coordinate regulation of glucose transporter function, number and gene expression by insulin and sulfonylureas in L6 rat skeletal muscle cell. J Clin Invest 1989;84:62–67.
35 Jacos DB, Hayes GR, Lockwood DH: In vitro effects of sulfonylurea on glucose transport and translocation of glucose transporters in adipocytes from streptozotocin-induced diabetic rats. Diabetes 1989;38:205–211.
36 Nyomba BL, Freymond D, Raz P, Stone K, Mott DM, Bogardus C: Skeletal muscle glycogen synthase activity in subjects with non-insulin-dependent diabetes mellitus after glyburide therapy. Metabolism 1990;39:1204–1210.
37 Grunberger G, Ryan J, Gordon Ph: Sulfonylureas do not affect insulin binding or glycaemic control in insulin-dependent diabetics. Diabetics 1982;31:890–891.
38 Ratzmann KP, Schultz B, Heinke P, Besch W: Tolbutamide does not alter insulin requirement in type 1 (insulin-dependent) diabetes. Diabetologia 1984;27:8–12.
39 Leblanc H, Thote A, Chatellier G, Passa Ph: Effet du glipizide sur le contrôle glycémique et la sensibilité périphérique à l'insuline chez les diabétiques de type 1. Diabete Metab 1990;16: 93–97.
40 Simonson D, Delprato S, Castellino P, Groop L, De Fronzo RA: Effect of glyburide on glycaemic control, insulin requirement and glucose metabolism in insulin-treated diabetic patients. Diabetes 1987;36:136–146.
41 Pernet A, Trimble ER, Kuntschen F, Assal JP, Kahn C, Renold AE: Sulfonylureas in insulin-dependent (type 1) diabetes evidence for an extrapancreatic effect in vivo. J Clin Endocrinol Metab 1985;61:247.
42 Garrel DR, Picq R, Bajard L, Harfouche M, Tourniaire J: Acute effect of glyburide on insulin sensitivity in type 1 diabetic patient. J Clin Endocrinol Metab 1987;65:896–900.
43 Ferner RE, Alberti KGMM, Rawlins MD: Massive glibenclamide overdose without hypoglycaemia in a man with diabetes after partial pancreatectomy. Hum Toxicol 1986;5:283–285.
44 Kirsch DM: Ciglitazone: A specific agent against type 2 post-receptor insulin resistance?; in Serrano-Rios M, Lefebvre PJ (eds): Diabetes 1985. Amsterdam, Elsevier, 1986, pp 824–830.

45 Fujiwara T, Yoshioka S, Yoskioka T, Ushiyama I, Horikoshi H: Characterization of new oral antidiabetic agent CS-045. Diabetes 1988;37:1549–1558.
46 Stevenson RW, Hutson NJ, Krupo MN, at al: Actions of novel antidiabetic agent englitazone in hyperglycaemic hyperinsulinemia ob/ob mice. Diabetes 1990;39:1218–1227.
47 Suter SL, Nolan JJ, Wallace P, Gumbiner B, Olefsky JM: Metabolic effects of new oral hypoglycemic agent C5-045 in NIDDM subjects. Diabetes Care 1992;15:193–203.
48 Brichard SM, Lederer J, Henquin JC: The insulin-like properties of vanadium: A curiosity on a perspective for the treatment of diabetes. Diabete Metab 1991;17:435–446.
49 Cros G, Mongold JJ, Serrano JJ, Ramanadham S, McNeill JH: Vanadium et diabète; in Journées de Diabétologie 1991. Paris, Flammarion, 1991, pp 193–201.
50 Meyerovitch J, Rothenberg P, Shechter Y, Bonner-Weir S, Kahn CR: Vanadate normalizes hyperglycaemia in two mouse models of non-insulin-dependent diabetes mellitus. J Clin Invest 1991;87:1286–1294.
51 Domingo JL, Gomel M, Llobet JM, Corbella J, Keen CL: Oral vanadium administration to streptozotocin-diabetic rats has marked negative side effects which are independent of the form of vanadium used. Toxicology 1991;66: 279–287.
52 Young JC, Treadway JL, Fader EI, Caslin RF: Effects of oral hypoglycaemic agent methylpalmoxyrate on exercise capacity of streptozotocin diabetic rats. Diabetes 1986;35:744–748.
53 Mandarino L, Tsalikian E, Barthold S, et al: Mechanism of hyperglycaemia and response to treatment with an inhibitor of fatty acid oxidation in a patient with insulin resistance due to anti-insulin receptor antibodies. J Clin Endocrinol Metab 1984;59:658–664.
54 Oellerich M, Haelkel R: Hydroxypropionic acid, a new class of hypoglycaemic substances. Horm Metab Res 1980;12:182–189.
55 Elias D, Rapoport M, Cohen IR, Shechter Y: Desensitization of the insulin receptor by anti-receptor antibodies in vivo is blocked by treatment of mice with β-adrenergic agonists. J Clin Invest 1988;81:1979–1988.
56 Ferre P, Penicaud L, Hitier Y, Meier M, Girard J: Hypoglycaemic effects of a β-agonist, Ro 16-8714 in streptozotocin diabetic rats. Decreased hepatic glucose production and increased glucose utilization in oxidative muscle. Metabolism 1992;41:180–183.
57 Quin JD, Fisher BM, Paterson KR, Inoue A, Beastall GH, MacCuish AC: Acute response to recombinant insulin-like growth factor 1 in a patient with Mendenhall's syndrome. N Engl J Med 1990;15:1425–1426.
58 Schoenle EJ, Zenobi PD, Torresani T, Werder EA, Zachmann M, Froesch ER: Recombinant human insulin-like growth factor-1 (rhIGF-1) reduces hyperglycaemia in patients with extreme insulin resistance. Diabetologia 1991;34: 675–679.

Horm Res 1992;38:57–61

Ph. De Nayer

Hormone and Metabolism Unit, International Institute of Cellular and Molecular Pathology (ICP), Nuclear Medicine and Clinical Chemistry Departments, University of Louvain Medical School, Brussels, Belgium

The Thyroid Hormone Receptors: Molecular Basis of Thyroid Hormone Resistance

Key Words

T_3 receptor
Thyroid hormone resistance
T_3 action

Abstract

Major progress has been achieved in the mechanism of action of thyroid hormones thanks to the identification of the T_3 receptor as the product of the proto-oncogene c-erbA. Recognition of subsets of receptors with and without T_3-binding properties and of the interaction of different receptors with each other leads to new insights in cell regulation and development. In thyroid hormone resistance, distinct mutations in the T_3-binding domain of thyroid hormone receptor (TR)β have been identified in unrelated families. No correlation between the type of mutation and tissue resistance has been established. Mutant TRs bind to thyroid hormone response elements (TREs) on both negative or positive T_3-controlled genes. Subjects with heterozygous TRβ gene deletion are not affected, supporting the hypothesis that mutant TRs act through a dominant negative effect. In generalized thyroid hormone resistance, mutated TRβ may interfere through competition for TREs and/or formation of inactive dimers. Finally, deficiency in T_3 receptor auxiliary protein or other accessory proteins or competition between mutant and normal TRs for these factors is not excluded.

Introduction

The interaction of thyroid hormones with a nuclear receptor represents the initial step of the effect of T_3 on gene expression. For more than two decades this receptor was known to be a DNA-binding protein but the lack of its availability in purified form has prevented the detailed analysis of its properties [1, 2].

A major breakthrough was provided in 1986 by the observation that the thyroid hormone receptor (TR) was the product of a proto-oncogene, c-erbA, the cellular homologue of v-erbA, involved in avian erythroblastosis. Two similar but not identical forms (α and β) of the receptor were identified, and accordingly they have been shown to be the product of two separate genes. The human TRα is coded by a gene on chromosome 17; the gene of TRβ is located on chromosome 3. The TRα shows a higher homology with the v-erbA protein than does the TRβ. The v-erbA protein does not bind T_3, probably due to a limited number of amino acid substitutions and deletions in the ligand-binding domain, whereas it is still able to bind to DNA [3–5].

Both the α and β forms are expressed albeit to a different extent in all tissues studied. The in vitro translated proteins of the cDNAs of TR bind T_3 with high affinity and other thyronines with affinities close to the nascent receptor [3, 4, 6]. The receptors bind to specific DNA sequences known as thyroid hormone response elements

Ph. De Nayer
Hormone and Metabolism Unit
International Institute of Cellular and Molecular Pathology (ICP)
Nuclear Medicine and Clinical Chemistry Departments
University of Louvain Medical School, B-1200 Brussels (Belgium)

0301–0163/92/0382–0057
$2.75/0

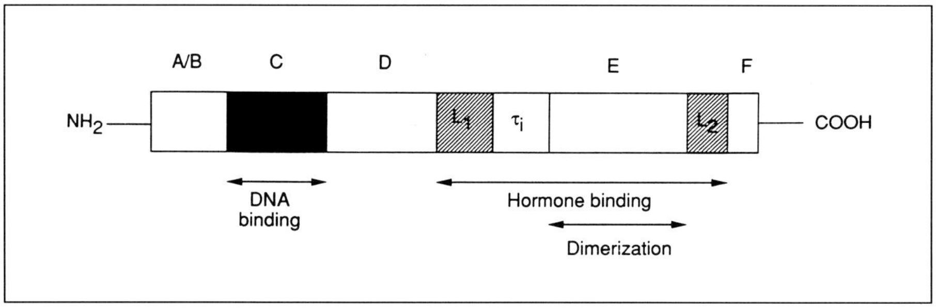

Fig. 1. Schematic representation of the TRβ, indicating the domains involved in DNA-binding (C), hormone-binding (E) trans-inactivating activity (τi) and dimerization.

(TREs) in the promotor region of thyroid hormone responsive gene. They have been shown to have the capacity to transactive target genes in transfection experiments [7–9]. The role of multiple TRs in cells remains unclear. The question may be raised whether they control the expression of specific genes in specific tissues.

The Structure of the Receptor

Sequence similarities among the receptors for steroids, thyronines, vitamin D_3, retinoic acid and other developmental hormones suggest that they belong to a receptor superfamily originating from an ancestral gene [10].

Distinct function-related regions have been recognized in these receptor proteins (fig. 1). The A/B region, located at the amino end, is probably involved in interactions with other proteins; the C region corresponds to the DNA-binding domain and contains two 'zinc fingers' recognizing the TRE's on the DNA, through amino acids in a Proximal box in finger 1 and in a Distal box in finger 2. No specific role is known for the D region. The E region at the carboxy-terminus is more complex: it contains a ligand-binding domain divided in two areas, a large area consisting of nine heptad repeats of hydrophobic amino acids as potential dimerization sites ('leucine zippers'), and a trans-inactivating region relieved by hormone binding (τi) [11–13].

T_3 Receptor Variants

Several isoforms of the receptors derived from various tissues in man and rat have been described. In addition to the active $TR\alpha_1$, variants originating from alternative splicing of the α gene primary transcripts have been identified in several tissues including heart and brain where they are present in high abundance [14–16]. These variants differ in length and amino acid sequence at the carboxy-terminus. These isoforms interact with the TREs but do not bind T_3. Nevertheless, they are named $TR\alpha_2$, α_3, ... or, better, c-erbAα_2 vI, vII ... The presence of a transcript from the opposite DNA strand of the α gene, generating a T_3 nonbinding T_3 'receptor', has also been reported (Rev-TRα or ear-1, for erbA-related protein). A regulatory mechanism exerted by this naturally occurring anti-sense RNA at the translational level has been suggested [17, 18]. Since both the T_3-binding and the T_3-nonbinding forms of the receptor may compete at the DNA-binding level, one is faced with the situation that within a given cell, the expression of the α genes may yield TRs with opposite effects. Interestingly, v-erbA may act in a similar way inasmuch as it does not bind T_3 but can bind to TREs [5, 19].

One isoform of the TRβ, the $TR\beta_2$, has been detected in the rat pituitary, and in discrete areas of the brain. It is identical to the $TR\beta_1$, except for divergences in length and amino acid sequence in the A/B domain. Interestingly, T_3 appears to decrease the density of the $TR\beta_2$ in the pituitary, suggesting a role of this receptor in the control of TSH gene expression [20–22].

Thyroid Hormone Response Element

The identification of TR-binding areas in the promotor region of target genes has led to the characterization of TREs with consensus sequences. The two half sites of TREs present in two typical configurations: as a palindrome (rGH) or as direct (tandem) repeats (myosin heavy chain) [7, 11]. Discrimination among specific DNA-binding sites is determined by three amino acids in the P box on the first Zn finger of the receptors. The glucocorticoid, mineralocorticoid, androgen and progesterone receptors all contain the same three discriminating amino acids (Gly, Ser, Val) and are able to recognize a same HRE. The

TR, RAR and the vitamin D receptor (VDR), as well as c-erbAα_2 and Rev-erbA-α, possess identical amino acids at the discriminatory site (Glu, Gly, Gly). Amino acids in the D box discriminate similar tandem repeats with distinct spacing (RARE, TRE, VDRE, ERE) [11, 13, 23, 24].

A nuclear protein, the T_3 receptor auxiliary protein (TRAP), enhances and stabilizes TR binding to TRE by interaction with a region in the hormone-binding domain and the TRE [25–27].

Dimers as a Model for Thyroid Hormone Nuclear Receptor

The presence of TRE half sites at the DNA-binding site and 'leucine zippers' in the ligand-binding domain support the hypothesis of dimerization of the receptor although the ability of TR to act via single half sites has not been excluded (fig. 2).

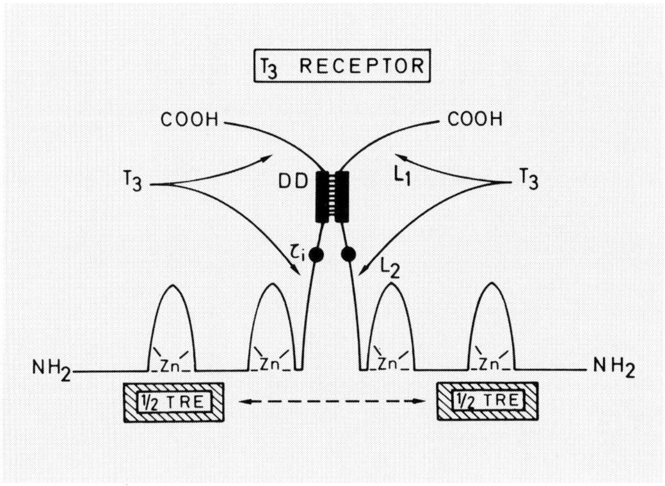

Fig. 2. Model for the dimerization of the TR.

This model would allow for the formation of receptor homodimers but also for heterodimers with other receptors such as RAR and VDR [7, 11, 12, 28, 29]. Along the same line, receptors with mutations in the T_3-binding domain may exert through dimerization a dominant negative activity on the receptor properties. Recent data however suggest that TR/TRAP heterodimers may be the stable complex occupying TREs in the presence of T_3 [30].

Molecular Defects of the TR in Thyroid Hormone Resistance

The hypothesis that thyroid hormone resistance is caused by abnormalities in the TR was only recently confirmed [31, 32]. Studies based on the analysis of restriction fragment length polymorphism (RFLP) have indicated that mutations in the TRβ cosegregated with thyroid hormone resistance [33–35]. Accordingly, base substitutions were observed in the T_3-binding domain of affected subjects. Interestingly, distinct mutations occurred in the different kindreds, with a clustering in the middle and carboxy-terminal regions of the hormone-binding domain [36–42]. In some families, two mutations have been found. Up to now, no mutation has been reported in the DNA-binding domain of the receptor. cDNA of mutants were cloned and the translation products analyzed for their binding properties: they showed reduced affinity for T_3 with a range extending from hardly detectable to near normal values; binding to TREs on positively (rat GH) or negatively (TSHβ) controlled genes was not affected [43–46]. These various mutations are not linked to specific phenotypes. Although base mutation appears the most frequent alteration in thyroid hormone resistance, Takeda et al. [47] have shown that in the first reported thyroid-resistant patient [48] another and surprising alteration was present. Indeed, this patient had a complete deletion of the T_3-binding and DNA-binding domains of the TRβ in both alleles. Heterozygous members for the deleted TRβ gene did not show either clinical or biochemical evidences for thyroid hormone resistance, suggesting in this type of alteration a recessive mode of inheritance. In addition, this observation leads to the conclusion that the TRβ gene does not appear to be essential for survival, and therefore that in the homozygous subjects hormone action would be mediated by the TRα. Yet another type of alteration has been reported: the deletion of a codon in the T_3-binding domain. The homozygous patient was severely affected, whereas in heterozygous members of this kindred, the mutant TRβ exerted a dominant negative control as in the case of single base mutation [49, 50] (table 1). The homozygous patient with codon deletion was more severely affected than the patient with homozygous TRβ deletion. This difference suggests that the mutant TRβ receptor may exert a dominant negative control of thyroid hormone effects mediated through TRα.

The molecular mechanism involved calls for a dominant negative inhibition by the mutant form on the wild

Table 1. Thyroid hormone resistance

TRβ alterations	Ref.
1. Mutations	36–42
Autosomal dominant	
Reported cases: heterozygous	
Number of kindreds = 28	
2. Gene deletion	47, 48
Autosomal recessive	
Reported cases heterozygous	
homozygous	
Number of kindreds = 1	
3. Codon deletion	49, 50
Autosomal dominant	
Reported cases heterozygous	
homozygous	
Number of kindreds = 1	

type. Indeed the complete deletion of one copy of the TRβ gene does not lead to thyroid hormone resistance. Accordingly, cotransfection experiments show that mutant TRβ can block the activity of TRα and TRβ [41, 44–46]. How this mechanism operates is still unclear: the mutant TRβ could compete for TRE or dimerize with wild type mutants to form inactive complexes. Hence variable degrees of thyroid hormone resistance would result from the relative concentration of mutant TRβ versus normal TR. A deficiency in the availability of TRAP or other factors may also possibly play a role.

Acknowledgement

The expert editorial assistance of Mrs. V. Henry is gratefully acknowledged.

References

1 Oppenheimer JH: The nuclear receptor-triiodothyronine complex: Relationship to thyroid hormone distribution, metabolism, and biological ation; in Oppenheimer JH, Samuels HH (eds): Molecular Basis of Thyroid Hormone Action. New York, Academic Press, 1983, pp 1–34.
2 De Nayer P: Thyroid hormone action at the cellular level. Hormone Res 1987;26:48–57.
3 Sap J, Munoz A, Damm K, Goldberg Y, Ghysdael J, Leutz A, Beug H, Vennström B: The c-erbA protein is a high-affinity receptor for thyroid hormone. Nature 1986;324:635–640.
4 Weinberger C, Thompson CP, Ong ES, Lebo R, Gruol DJ: The c-erbA gene encodes a thyroid hormone receptor. Nature 1986;324:641–646.
5 Beug H, Vennström B: Avian erythroleukaemia: Possible mechanisms involved in v-erbA oncogene function; in Parker MG (ed): Nuclear Hormone Receptors. New York, Academic Press, 1991, pp 355–375.
6 Putlitz zu J, Datta S, Madison LD, Macchia E, Jameson JL: Human thyroid hormone β_1-receptor produced by recombinant baculovirus-infected insect cells. Biochem Biophys Res Commun 1991;175:285–290.
7 Glass CK, Holloway JM: Regulation of gene expression by the thyroid hormone receptor. Biochim Biophys Acta 1990;1032:157–176.
8 Brent GA, Moore DD, Larsen RP: Thyroid hormone regulation of gene expression. Annu Rev Physiol 1991;51:17–35.
9 Chin WW: Nuclear hormone receptors; in Parker MG (ed): Nuclear Hormone Receptors. New York, Academic Press, 1991, pp 79–102.
10 Evans RM: The steroid and thyroid hormone receptor superfamily. Science 1988;240:889–895.
11 Forman BM, Samuels HH: Dimerization among nuclear hormone receptors. New Biol 1990;2:587–594.
12 Forman BM, Yang CR, Au M, Casanova J, Ghysdael J, Samuels HH: A domain containing leucine-zipper-like motifs mediate novel in vivo interactions between the thyroid hormone and retinoic acid receptors. Mol Endocrinol 1989;3:1610–1626.
13 Umesono K, Evans RM: Determinants of target gene specificity for steroid/thyroid hormone receptors. Cell 1989;57:1139–1146.
14 Koenig RJ, Lazar MA, Hodin RA, Brent GA, Larsen RP, Chin WW, Moore DD: Inhibition of thyroid hormone action by a non-hormone binding c-erbA protein generated by alternative mRNA splicing. Nature 1989;337:659–661.
15 Izumo S, Mahdavi V: Thyroid hormone receptor α isoforms generated by alternative splicing differentially activate myosin HC gene transcription. Nature 1988;334:539–542.
16 Mitsuhashi T, Tennyson GE, Nikodem VM: Alternative splicing generates messages encoding rat c-erbA proteins that do not bind thyroid hormone. Proc Natl Acad Sci USA 1988;85:5804–5808.
17 Lazar MA, Jones KE, Chin WW: Isolation of a cDNA encoding human rev-erbAα: Transcription from the non-coding DNA strand of a thyroid hormone receptor gene results in a related protein which does not bind thyroid hormone. DNA Cell Biol 1990;9:77–83.
18 Markham BE, Tsika RW, Bahl JJ, Anderson PG, Morkin E: An anti-sense c-erbA clone inhibits thyroid hormone-induced expression from the α-myosin heavy chain promoter. J Biol Chem 1990;265:6489–6493.
19 Damm K, Thompson C, Evans RM: Protein encoded by v-erbA functions as a thyroid-hormone receptor antagonist. Nature 1989;339:593–597.
20 Hodin RA, Lazar MA, Wintman BI, Darling DS, Koenig RJ, Larsen RP, Moore DD, Chin WW: Identification of a thyroid hormone receptor that is pituitary-specific. Science 1989;244:76–79.
21 Cook CC, Kakucska I, Lechan RM, Koenig RJ: Expression of thyroid hormone receptor β_2 in rat hypothalamus. Endocrinology 1992;130:1077–1079.
22 Childs GV, Taub K, Jones KE, Chin WW: Triiodothyronine receptor β_2 messenger ribonucleic acid expression by somatotropes and thyrotropes: Effect of propylthiouracil-induced hypothyroidism in rats. Endocrinology 1991;129:2767–2773.
23 Umesono K, Giguere V, Glass CK, Rosenfeld MG, Evans RM: Retinoic acid and thyroid hormone induce gene expression through a common responsive element. Nature 1988;336:1262–1265.
24 Umesono K, Murakami KK, Thompson CC, Evans RM: Direct repeats as selective response elements for the thyroid hormone, retinoic acid and vitamin D_3 receptors. Cell 1991;65:1255–1266.

25 Murray MB, Towle HC: Identification of nuclear factors that enhance binding of the thyroid hormone receptor to a thyroid hormone response element. Mol Endocrinol 1989;3; 1434-1442.

26 Beebe JS, Darling DS, Chin WW: 3,5,3′-Triiodothyronine receptor auxiliary protein (TRAP) enhances receptor binding by interactions within the thyroid hormone response element. Mol Endocrinol 1991;5:85–93.

27 Yen PM, Darling DS, Chin WW: Basal and thyroid hormone receptor auxiliary protein-enhanced binding of thyroid hormone receptor isoforms to native thyroid hormone response elements. Endocrinology 1991;129:3331–3336.

28 Glass CK, Lipkin SM, Devary OV, Rosenfeld MG: Positive and negative regulation of gene transcription by a retinoic acid-thyroid hormone receptor heterodimer. Cell 1989;59:697–708.

29 Glass CK, Direnzo J, Kurokawa R, Han Z: Regulation of gene expression by retinoic acid receptors. DNA Cell Biol 1991;10:623–638.

30 Yen PM, Darling DS, Carter RL, Forgione M, Umeda PK, Chin WW: Triiodothyronine (T_3) decreases binding to DNA by T_3-receptor homodimers but not auxiliary protein heterodimers. J Biol Chem 1992;267:3665–3568.

31 Refetoff S: Syndromes of thyroid hormone resistance. Am J Physiol 1982;243:E88–98.

32 Daubresse JC, Dozin-Vanroye B, De Nayer Ph, De Visscher M: Partial resistance to thyroid hormones: Reduced affinity of lymphocyte nuclear receptors for T_3 in two siblings; in Stockigt JR, Nagataki S (eds): Thyroid Research. VIII. Canberra, Australian Academy of Science, 1980, pp 295–298.

33 Usala SJ, Bale AE, Gesundheit N, Weinberger C, Lash RW, Wondisford FE, McBride OW, Weintraub BD: Tight linkage between the syndrome of generalized thyroid hormone resistance and the human c-erbAβ gene. Mol Endocrinol 1988;2:1217–1220.

34 Fein HG, Burman KD, Djuh YY, Usala SJ, Bale AE, Weintraub BD, Smallridge RC. Tight linkage of the human c-erbAβ gene with the syndrome of generalized thyroid hormone resistance is present in multiple kindreds. J Endocrinol Invest 1991;14:219–223.

35 Usala SJ, Weintraub BD: Thyroid hormone resistance syndromes. Trends Endocrinol Metab 1991;2:140–144.

36 Sakurai A, Takeda K, Ain K, Ceccarelli P, Nakai A, Seino S, Bell GL, Refetoff S, De Groot LJ: Generalized resistance to thyroid hormone associated with a mutation in the ligand-binding domain of the human thyroid hormone receptor β. Proc Natl Acad Sci USA 1989;86:8977–8981.

37 Takada K, Balzano S, Sakurai A, De Groot LJ, Refetoff S: Screening of nineteen unrelated families with generalized resistance to thyroid hormone for known mutations in the thyroid hormone receptor β gene and the detection of a new mutation. J Clin Invest 1991;87:496–502.

38 Usala SJ, Menke JB, Watson TL, Berard J, Bradley WEC, Bale AE, Lash RW, Weintraub BD: A new point mutation in the 3,5,3′-triiodothyronine-binding domain of the c-erbAβ thyroid hormone receptor is tightly linked to generalized thyroid hormone resistance. J Clin Endocrinol Metab 1991;72:32–38.

39 Parrilla R, Mixson AJ, McPherson JA, McClaskey JH, Weintraub BD: Characterization of seven novel mutations of the c-erbAβ gene in unrelated kindreds with generalized thyroid hormone resistance. Evidence for two 'hot spot' regions of the ligand binding domain. J Clin Invest 1991;88:2123–2130.

40 Takeda K, Weiss RE, Refetoff S: Rapid localization of mutations in the thyroid hormone receptor-β gene by denaturing gradient gel electrophoresis in 18 families with thyroid hormone resistance. J Clin Endocrinol Metab 1992;74:712–719.

41 Adams M, Nagaya T, Tone Y, Jameson JL, Chatterjee VKK: Functional properties of a novel mutant thyroid hormone receptor in a family with generalized thyroid hormone resistance syndrome. Clin Endocrinol 1992;36: 281–289.

42 Usala SJ, Tennyson GE, Bale AE, Lash RW, Gesundheit N, Wondisford FE, Accili D, Hauser P, Weintraub BD: A base mutation of the c-erbAβ thyroid hormone receptor in a kindred with generalized thyroid hormone resistance. Molecular heterogeneity in two other kindreds. J Clin Invest 1990;85:93–100.

43 Usala JS, Wondisford FE, Watson TL, Menke JB, Weintraub BD: Thyroid hormone and DNA binding properties of a mutant c-erbAβ receptor associated with generalized thyroid hormone resistance. Biochem Biophys Res Commun 1990;171:575–580.

44 Sakurai A, Miyamoto T, Refetoff S, De Groot LJ: Dominant negative transcriptional regulation by a mutant thyroid hormone receptor β in a family with generalized resistance to thyroid hormone. Mol Endocrinol 1990;4:1988–1994.

45 Chatterjee VKK, Nagaya T, Madison LD, Datta S, Rentoumis A, Jameson JL: Thyroid hormone resistance syndrome. Inhibition of normal receptor function by mutant thyroid hormone receptors. J Clin Invest 1991;87: 1977–1984.

46 Meier CA, Dickstein BM, Ashizawa K, McClaskey JH, Muchmore P, Ransom SC, Menke JB, Had EH, Usala SJ, Bercu BB, Cheng SY, Weintraub BD: Variable transcriptional activity and ligand binding of mutant β_1 3,5,3′-triiodothyronine receptors from four families with generalized resistance to thyroid hormone. Mol Endocrinol 1992;6:248–258.

47 Takeda K, Sakurai A, De Groot LJ, Refetoff S: Recessive inheritance of thyroid hormone resistance caused by complete deletion of the protein-coding region of the thyroid hormone receptor-β gene. J Clin Endocrinol Metab 1992;74:49–55.

48 Refetoff S, De Wind LT, De Groot LJ: Familial syndrome combining deaf-mutism, stippled epiphyses, goiter, and abnormally high PBI: Possible target organ refractoriness to thyroid hormone. J Clin Endocrinol Metab 1967;27: 279–294.

49 Ono S, Schwartz ID, Mueller TD, Root AW, Usala SJ, Bercu BB: Homozygosity for a dominant negative thyroid hormone receptor gene responsible for generalized resistance to thyroid hormone. J Clin Endocrinol Metab 1991; 73:990–994.

50 Usala SJ, Menke JB, Watson TL, Wondisford FE, Weintraub BD, Berard J, Bradley WEC, Ono S, Mueller OT, Bercu BB. A homozygous deletion in the c-erbAβ thyroid hormone receptor gene in a patient with generalized thyroid hormone resistance: Isolation and characterization of the mutant receptor. Mol Endocrinol 1991;5:327–335.

Horm Res 1992;38:62–65

C. Jaffiol[a]
F. de Boisvilliers[a]
L. Baldet[a]
J. Torresani[b]

[a] Service d'Endocrinologie, Hôpital Lapeyronie, Montpellier;
[b] Biochimie Médicale, Faculté de Médecine, INSERM U38, Marseille, France

Thyroid Hormone Generalized Resistance

Key Words
Thyroid hormone
Resistance
Goiter

Abstract
The syndromes of thyroid hormone resistance may affect overall or only some tissues. The generalized resistance is an inherited disease which involves a familial eumetabolic or hypometabolic goiter, increased free thyroid hormones with normal or elevated plasma TSH levels; children may present mental retardation, deafness, short stature and delayed bone age. The disease is frequently misdiagnosed. In vivo and in vitro tests may be used to assess the diagnosis. The defect of increment of sex hormone-binding globulin after administration of T_3 may be useful in the demonstration of the disease. Therapy uses high T_4 or T_3 doses in hypometabolic patients. The generalized thyroid hormone resistance could be linked to abnormalities at the T_3 receptor and c-erb A gene level, as a consequence of different point mutations or deletions involving the hormone-binding domain.

Resistance to thyroid hormone can be defined as the impaired response of target tissues to an adequate provision of the hormone [1]. The syndrome of generalized resistance to thyroid hormone (GRTH), described in 1967 by Refetoff et al. [2], is characterized by elevated serum levels of free thyroid hormones with inappropriately normal or elevated thyrotropin (TSH).

Epidemiology

Up until 1990, 196 affected subjects had been reported, most of them after 1981, of which 181 were familial (47 families) [3]. Men and women are similarly affected without ethnic or geographical differences. In most subjects, the disorder has been inherited as an autosomal-dominant trait with variability in tissue responsiveness to elevated thyroid hormones. However, recessive transmission was found in about 10% of families with proven or suspected consanguinity in four or five [4, 5].

Clinical and Biological Features

The syndrome is rarely diagnosed at birth and is more often recognized in infancy and adult life. The cardinal features of GRTH are elevated serum levels of free T_4 and T_3, nonsuppressed thyrotropin level with a preserved response to protirelin (TRH), absence of the usual symptoms and metabolic consequences of thyroid hormone excess and goiter [1]. Although the apparent resistance to thyroid hormone varies in severity, it is always partial, probably because a complete defect would be incompatible with life.

Clinical Features

Clinical features involve a familial homogeneous or nodular goiter, present at an early age, recurring after partial thyroidectomy. Most of the patients are eumetabolic. However, children may present symptoms of hypothyroidism with deafness, short stature, delayed bone development, stippled epiphysis, school retardation [2]. Para-

C. Jaffiol
Service d'Endocrinologie
Hôpital Lapeyronie
F–34059 Montpellier Cedex (France)

0301–0163/92/0382–0062
$2.75/0

doxically, some patients may present hyperactivity or tachycardia suggestive of hyperthyroidism leading to the notion that the sensitivity to thyroid hormone varies in different organs. There is a wide spectrum of refractoriness to thyroid hormone action among different tissues; patients with GRTH in different kindreds present with variable patterns of tissue resistance [6, 7]. In many subjects, a long-standing enlargement of the thyroid gland represents the sole abnormality on clinical examination.

Reduction of the serum thyroid hormone levels towards normal by thyroid surgery, radioiodide or antithyroid drugs, increases serum TSH concentration and may induce overt symptoms of thyroid hormone deficiency.

Biological Abnormalities

The syndrome may be suspected when thyroid hormone levels are found to be elevated in association with nonsuppressed TSH.

The concentration and the production rate of total and free thyroid hormones are increased. Their molecular structure, transport and peripheral metabolism are normal [1] and circulating inhibitors are absent.

The basal levels of TSH are usually in a normal range or moderately elevated [1] with normal response to TRH and metoclopramide. Suppression of TSH can be obtained with dopamine, bromocriptine, triiodothyroacetic acid and high doses of T_3 [8]. The αTSH/TSH ratio is normal. Basal and stimulated or suppressed values of prolactin are unmodified [9].

The resistance of target tissues to thyroid hormone can be assessed in vivo with the failure of T_3 to induce metabolic responses in peripheral tissues. Peripheral markers of thyroid hormone action including basal metabolic rate, cardiac contractility, deep tendon reflex relaxation time, sleeping pulse rate, sex hormone-binding globulin (SHBG), ferritin, angiotensin-converting enzyme, cholesterol, carotene, creatine phosphokinase in serum, hydroxyproline, carnitine, creatinine, magnesium, urea nitrogen and AMPc in urine remain in a normal range. It is imperative to compare values obtained in the same individual before and during the administration of graded doses of thyroid hormone rather than to interpret baseline data on the basis of normal values [7]. In vitro, T_3 does not increase low density lipoprotein (LDL) degradation [10] and does not reduce glycosaminoglycan synthesis [11] or fibronectin synthesis [12] in skin fibroblasts of subjects with GRTH.

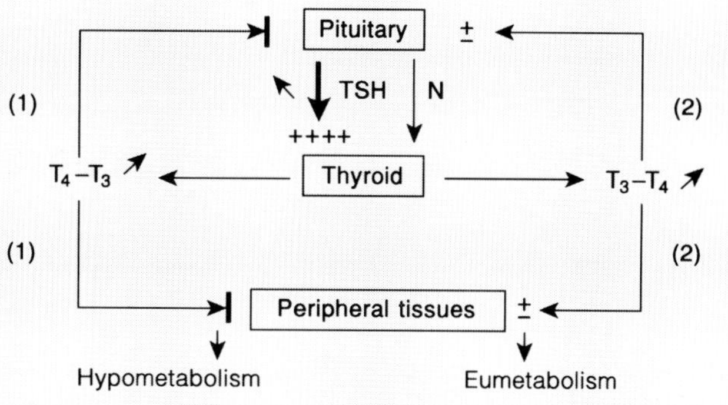

Fig. 1. The variations of sensitivity of pituitary and peripheral tissues to thyroid hormone (■ = total inhibition ± partial inhibition of thyroid hormone action) may explain the large spectrum of clinical aspects of GRTH.

Table 1. Main causes of detectable TSH in plasma despite raised free thyroid hormones

Familial dysalbuminemic hyperthyroxinemia
T_4-T_3 antibodies – TSH antibodies
Inadequate T_4 substitutive therapy of hypothyroidism
Inappropriate TSH secretion
TSH-producing tumor
Thyroid hormone resistance

Diagnosis

GRTH is frequently misdiagnosed [13]. It is exceptionally detected at birth by screening tests for neonatal diagnosis of hypothyroidism [3]. In adults, a familial goiter remains frequently the sole manifestation of the disease.

An elevation of free T_3 and T_4, with a nonsuppressed TSH, should easily eliminate congenital abnormalities in protein-binding globulin. Acquired and familial thyroxin-binding globulin excess rise total thyroid hormones but free hormone levels remain in the normal range. Acquired and familial increase in TBPA concentration, altered T_4 binding to albumin in subjects with familial hyperthyroxinemic dysalbuminemia or the presence of circulating antibodies to T_4, T_3 or TSH may increase free thyroid hormone levels but none of these conditions cause thyroid gland enlargement and all can be recognized by specific tests [1, 14]. More difficult is to distinguish GRTH and

Table 2. Generalized thyroid hormone resistance pathophysiology

Large deletion in the β receptor gene
Point mutations (n deletion) in the β receptor gene
– Amino acid substitutions in the thyroid hormone-binding domain of the receptor
– Inhibitory activity of mutant receptors (dominant negative action)
Inactive dimers
Competition for binding to DNA or to other transcription factors

the two conditions of TSH-induced hyperthyroidism: pituitary resistance to thyroid hormone and TSH producing pituitary adenoma. In these cases, SHBG seems to be useful to differentiate the neoplasic form of inappropriate secretion of thyrotropin with resistance to thyroid hormone [15].

However, Graves' disease is the most common error of diagnosis due to the presence of a goiter associated with increased plasma free T_3-T_4 and, in some patients, hyperactivity and tachycardia. The ratio of serum T_3/T_4 remains in the normal range contrary to the majority of untreated patients with hyperthyroidism. In all these cases the presence of a normal or increased circulating TSH is the best argument against chronic causes of hyperthyroidism.

Therapy

In most cases, no treatment is required and the partial resistance to thyroid hormone is compensated with the increment in endogenous thyroid hormones [1]. In other cases, when hypometabolism is present, high doses of exogenous T_4 (500–1,000 μg daily) or T_3 (200–400 μg daily) are required. In such instances, judicious administration of supraphysiologic doses of hormone is indicated. It should be individually determined by assessing the peripheral tissue responses [16]. TSH evaluation and peripheral markers are assessed. Growth and mental development can be evaluated in children. Development of a catabolic state is observed in overtreated subjects.

Physiopathology

Soon after the description of the syndrome, it was postulated that the defect resides at the genetic level and that it is most likely caused by abnormal thyroid hormone receptor. The binding of T_3 to nuclear thyroid hormone receptor has been reported either decreased or normal [14].

Determination of amino acid sequence of the human c-erb A β thyroid hormone receptor, deduced from cDNA sequencing, has enabled evaluation of the genetic basis for GRTH. Four main isoforms of the thyroid hormone receptor so far identified (c-erb A α_1 and α_2; c-erb A β_1 and β_2) are generated by alternative splicing of primary transcripts of two c-erb A genes (α and β) located on human chromosome 17 and 3 respectively [17]. With the exception of the α_2 isoform, the other three forms bind thyroid hormone and function as thyroid hormone receptor. The α and β receptors present overlapping and variable, regulated, tissue distribution; in some cases, the receptors are expressed in distinct populations of cells, even within a given tissue. This can explain the paucity of abnormalities in most of the T_3-binding studies. A genetic linkage between the β gene and the syndrome of GRTH has been described [6] in several families.

Different point mutations in the ligand-binding domain of one allele of the β gene have been described in unrelated families with GRTH and also a large and a small deletion [4, 6, 18, 19]. Two of the three mutations first described and the small deletion resulted in decreased receptor affinity for T_3.

Direct sequencing of PCR amplified genomic DNA [17] and denaturing gradient gel electrophoresis of amplified DNA fragments from 5 exons of the β gene [20] have identified about 23 novel mutations, all in the ligand-binding domain of the T_3 receptor with two 'hot spots'. These mutations (most of them single-base substitution) are clustered in the middle and carboxyl terminal regions of the T_3-binding domain (exons 7 and 8) and appear to cause amino acid substitution. For certain amino acids, more than one type of mutation has been described in different kindreds. Moreover, three families have more than one base substitution in the β receptor [20]. Some mutant β receptors produced in vitro were found to bind T_3 with reduced affinity and were also found to be functionally deficient and to impair the activity of normal receptors in transient gene expression assays. This provided hypothesis for the dominant mode of inheritance of the GRTH syndrome [21].

The large deletion that involves the whole DNA- and T_3-binding domain in both alleles of the β gene is responsible for the recessive inheritance of the syndrome described in the initial kindred [2, 22]. In these cases, survival and maintenance of an euthyroid state are presumably mediated through expression of the thyroid hormone receptor α gene present in affected subjects and the maintenance of high thyroid hormone levels. Based on this observation, deletion on one allele of the β receptor gene is not sufficient to cause thyroid hormone resistance since the heterozygotes are normal.

Another case of homozygosity has been reported to be responsible for a more severe form of GRTH and it is interesting to note that in this family, heterozygotes also have the syndrome [23]. The clinical differences in these patients indicate that a dominant negative form of β receptor can inhibit at least some thyroid hormone action mediated by the α receptor.

There is considerable evolution in the understanding of the syndrome of GRTH and the recent progress in characterization of distinct topographic clustering of mutations provides an invaluable tool for the molecular dissection of thyroid receptor function [17].

References

1 Refetoff S: The syndrome of generalized resistance to thyroid hormone. Endocrine Res 1989;15:717–743.
2 Refetoff S, De Wind LT, Degroot LJ: Familial syndrome combining deaf-mutism, stippled epiphysis, goiter and abnormally high PBI possible target organ refractoriness to thyroid hormone. J Clin Endocrinol 1967;27:279–294.
3 Weiss RE, Balzano S, Scherberg NH, Refetoff S: Neonatal detection of generalized resistance to thyroid hormone. JAMA 1990;264:2245–2250.
4 Takeda S, Balzano S, Sakurai A, Degroot LJ, Refetoff S: Screening of nineteen unrelated families with generalized resistance to thyroid hormone receptor β gene and the detection of a new mutation. J Clin Invest 1991;87:496–502.
5 Refetoff S: Resistance to thyroid hormone revisited. Thyroid Today 1990;13:1–11.
6 Usula SJ, Menke JB, Watson TL, Berard J, Edward W, Bradley C, Bale AE, Lash RW, Weintraub BD: A new point mutation in the 3,5,3′-triiodothyronine binding domain of the C erb A thyroid hormone receptor is tightly linked to generalized thyroid hormone resistance. J Clin Endocrinol Metab 1991;72:32–38.
7 Smallridge RC, Parker RA, Wiggs EA, Rajagopal KR, Fein HG: Thyroid hormone resistance in a large kindred: Physiologic, biochemical, pharmacologic and neuropsychologic studies. Am J Med 1989;86:289–296.
8 Wemeau JL: Les syndromes de résistance et d'hypersensibilité aux hormones thyroidiennes. Sem Hôp Paris 1989;65:1325–1330.
9 Sarne DH, Sobieszczyk S, Ain KB, Refetoff S: Serum thyrotropin and prolactin in the syndrome of generalized resistance to thyroid hormone: Responses to thyrotropin-releasing hormone stimulation and short-term triiodothyronine suppression. J Clin Endocrinol Metab 1990;70;1305–1311.
10 Chait A, Kanter R, Green W, Kenny M: Defective thyroid hormone action in fibroblasts cultured from subjects with the syndrome of resistance to thyroid hormone. J Clin Endocrinol Metab 1982;54:767–772.
11 Murata Y, Refetoff S, Horwitz AL, Smith TJ: Hormonal regulation of glycosaminoglycan accumulation in fibroblasts from patients with resistance to thyroid hormone. J Clin Endocrinol Metab 1983;57:1233–1239.
12 Ceccarelli P, Refetoff S, Murata Y: Resistance to thyroid hormone diagnosed by the reduced response of fibroblasts to the triiodothyronine-induced suppression of fibronectin synthesis. J Clin Endocrinol Metab 1987;65:242–246.
13 Hopwood NJ, Sauder SE, Shapiro B, Sisson JC: Familial partial peripheral and pituitary resistance to thyroid hormone: A frequently missed diagnosis? Pediatrics 1986;78:1114–1122.
14 Franklyn JA: Syndromes of thyroid hormone resistance. Clin Endocrinol 1991;34:237–245.
15 Beck-Peccoz P, Roncoroni R, Mariotti S, Medri G, Marcocci C, Brabant G, Forloni F, Pinchera A, Faglia G: Sex hormone-binding globulin measurement in patients with inappropriate secretion of thyrotropin (IST): Evidence against selective pituitary thyroid hormone resistance in nonneoplasic IST. J Clin Endocrinol Metab 1990;70:19–25.
16 Sarne DH, Refetoff S, Rosenfield RL, Farriaux JP: Sex hormone binding globulin in the diagnosis of peripheral tissue resistance to thyroid hormone: The value of changes after short-term triiodothyronine administration. J Clin Endocrinol Metab 1988;66:740–746.
17 Parilla R, Mixson AJ, McPherson JA, McClaskey JH, Weintraub BD: Characterization of seven novel mutations of the c-erb A β gene in unrelated kindreds with generalized thyroid hormone resistance. Evidence of two 'hot spot' regions of the ligand-binding domain. J Clin Invest 1991;88:2123–2130.
18 Usala SJ, Tennyson GE, Bale AE, Lash RW, Gesundheit N, Wondisford FE, Accili D, Hauser P, Weintraub BD: A base mutation of the C erb A thyroid hormone receptor in a kindred with generalized thyroid hormone resistance. J Clin Invest 1990;85:93–100.
19 Sakurai A, Takeda K, Ain K, Ceccarelli P, Nakai A, Seino S, Bell GI, Refetoff S, De Groot JL: Generalized resistance to thyroid hormone associated with a mutation in the ligand-binding domain of the human thyroid hormone receptor. Proc Natl Acad Sci USA 1989;86:8977–8981.
20 Takeda K, Weiss RE, Refetoff S: Rapid localization of mutations in the thyroid hormone receptor β gene by denaturing gradient gel electrophoresis in 18 families with thyroid hormone resistance. J Clin Endocrinol Metab 1992;74:712–719.
21 Chatterjee KKK, Nagaya T, Maddison LD, Datta S, Rentoumis A, Jameson JL: Thyroid hormone resistance syndrome. Inhibition of normal receptor function by mutant thyroid hormone receptors. J Clin Invest 1991;87:1977–1984.
22 Takeda K, Sakurai A, De Groot LJ, Refetoff S: Recessive inheritance of thyroid hormone resistance caused by complete deletion of the protein-coding region of the thyroid hormone receptor β gene. J Clin Endocrinol Metab 1992;74:49–55.
23 Ono S, Schwartz ID, Mueller OT, Root AW, Usala SJ, Bercu BB: Homozygosity for a dominant negative thyroid hormone receptor gene responsible for generalized resistance to thyroid hormone. J Clin Endocrinol Metab 1991;73:990–994.

Horm Res 1992;38:66–72

P. Beck-Peccoz
F. Forloni
D. Cortelazzi
L. Persani
M.-J. Papandreou
C. Asteria
G. Faglia

Institute of Endocrine Sciences, University of Milan, Ospedale Maggiore IRCCS, Milan, Italy

Pituitary Resistance to Thyroid Hormones

Key Words
Resistance to thyroid hormones
Pituitary resistance
Generalized resistance
Hyperthyroidism
Thyroid hormone receptors
Thyroid hormone analogs
T_3 receptor mutations

Abstract
Pituitary thyroid hormone resistance (PRTH) refers to a particular form of thyroid hormone refractoriness that is accompanied by peripheral hyperthyroidism, as only the TSH-secreting pituitary cells appear to be resistant to the effects of thyroid hormones. The presence of PRTH is suspected and diagnosed on the basis of the finding of high free thyroid hormone levels along with unsuppressed TSH, clinical signs and symptoms of hyperthyroidism and values of at least one of the parameters evaluating peripheral thyroid hormone action in the hyperthyroid range. However, most patients with PRTH present with clinical signs and symptoms of thyroid dysfunction, particularly goiter and tachycardia, overlapping those recorded in patients with generalized thyroid hormone resistance (GRTH), i.e. refractoriness to thyroid hormones at both pituitary and peripheral tissue level. Moreover, most of them display normal values of other parameters evaluating the peripheral effects of thyroid hormones and bear mutations in the gene encoding for T_3 nuclear receptors similar to those found in patients with GRTH. These findings are questioning the existence of PRTH as a separate clinical entity and support the view that the various forms of thyroid hormone resistance may be part of a spectrum of disease with variable expression in different issues.

Introduction

In 1967, Refetoff et al. [1–3] first discovered a syndrome characterized by reduced response of target tissues to high levels of circulating thyroid hormones. The syndrome was accompanied by clinical signs and symptoms of hypothyroidism and was called generalized resistance to thyroid hormone action (GRTH). A few years later, a patient with the same biochemical features of GRTH patients, i.e. elevated levels of circulating free thyroid hormones in the presence of unsuppressed TSH concentrations, but peripheral stigmata of hyperthyroidism, was described by Gershengorn and Weintraub [4]. Moreover, the measurement of some parameters of peripheral thyroid hormone action showed values in the hyperthyroid range, a fact that further supported the presence of a normal response of the peripheral tissues to high levels of circulating thyroid hormones. This form of thyroid hormone

Paolo Beck-Peccoz, MD
Institute of Endocrine Sciences, University of Milan
Ospedale Maggiore IRCCS
Via F. Sforza, 35
I-20122 Milano (Italy)

0301–0163/92/0382–0066
$2.75/0

refractoriness was named 'selective' pituitary resistance to thyroid hormones (PRTH) or, alternatively, central hyperthyroidism due to nonneoplastic inappropriate secretion of TSH, being the neoplastic form due to the presence of TSH-secreting pituitary adenomas [5, 6]. PRTH was subsequently described in several additional patients and families [7], though the differential diagnosis with GRTH was in most instances very difficult, as the clinical signs and symptoms of thyrotoxicosis in a given patient are often vague and subjective, and the parameters to gauge thyroid hormone action are limited and somewhat qualitative [8]. Indeed, recent study on sex hormone-binding globulin (SHBG) measurement, taken as one of the best parameters to gauge the peripheral thyroid hormone effects, demonstrated that all the 15 tested patients with PRTH had normal levels of SHBG [9]. Therefore, it was concluded that the resistance to thyroid hormone in patients with PRTH does not appear 'selective' at the pituitary level, but also does involve at least the hepatic cells synthesizing and secreting SHBG. Furthermore, recent studies on the gene encoding for thyroid hormone receptors whose alterations are responsible for the thyroid hormone resistance [10–18], indicated that patients with similar genetic defects may display different phenotypic appearance of the disease [3, 5, 19].

The present review will focus on the current pitfalls which may be encountered in making the diagnosis of PRTH.

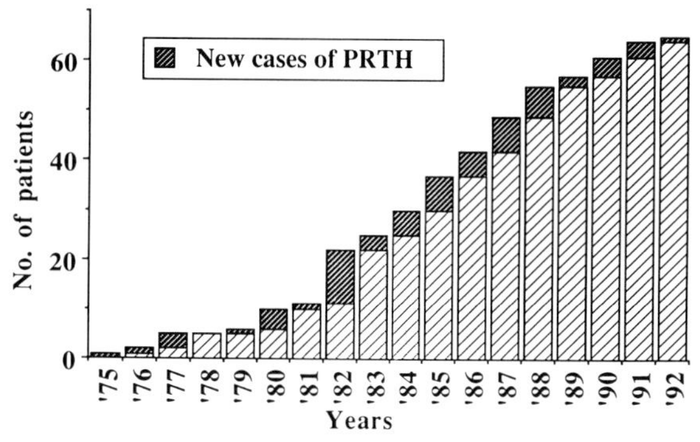

Fig. 1. Total number and incidence of new cases per year of patients with PRTH recorded in the literature until April 1992.

Occurrence and Diagnosis of PRTH

PRTH is a very rare disease, up to now reported in only 65 patients (fig. 1) [7]. The presence of PRTH was suspected and diagnosed on the basis of the finding of high free thyroid hormone levels along with unsuppressed TSH, clinical signs and symptoms of hyperthyroidism and, in some instances, values of at least one parameter of peripheral thyroid hormone action in the range of hyperthyroidism [5, 6, 9]. The number of reported cases will probably increase in the next years with the more wide use of the ultrasensitive immunometric assays for TSH measurement. Contrary to previous radioimmunoassays (RIAs), these methods allow a clear distinction between hyperthyroid patients (in whom TSH secretion is suppressed) and euthyroid subjects (in whom TSH secretion is not suppressed) and, therefore, they are used as first-line test for the evaluation of the thyroid function.

Based on the finding of measurable serum TSH levels in the presence of elevated thyroid hormone concentrations, several patients previously thought to be affected with Graves' disease could be correctly classified as bearing an inappropriate secretion of TSH due to thyroid hormone resistance or to a TSH-secreting pituitary adenoma. As far as the presence of TSH-secreting pituitary adenoma is concerned, patients with this rare type of pituitary tumor may be easily distinguished from those with PRTH or GRTH on the basis of the following findings: (a) presence of specific lesions at the sella turcica imaging (MRI, high resolution CT scan) [6, 20]; (b) high circulating levels of glycoprotein hormone α-subunit (α-SU) and elevated α-SU/TSH molar ratio [21]; (c) absent or impaired TSH responses to both stimulatory and inhibitory tests, and (d) values of parameters evaluating iodothyronine effects on peripheral tissues, such as SHBG, in the hyperthyroid range [9].

Clinical Features and Biochemical Findings

The analysis of all reported cases of PRTH indicates that the disease becomes clinically apparent and at any age, as in patients with GRTH (table 1). The distribution between sexes shows a female:male ratio of 2:1 in PRTH, while it is about 1:1 in GRTH. In most patients with PRTH, the disease appears to be sporadic, while the majority of patients with GRTH had at least another affected member of the family (table 1). However, in our experience, the incidence of familial cases is about 90% in both PRTH and GRTH.

About two-thirds of patients with PRTH and more than half of those with GRTH presented with a long medical history of thyroid dysfunction, misdiagnosed as

Graves' disease and inappropriately treated with thyroidectomy and/or radioiodine administration. In fact, some clinical features of hyperthyroidism, particularly goiter and tachycardia, are present both in resistant and in Graves' patients (table 1). Nonetheless, bilateral or monolateral exophthalmos has never been reported in resistant patients, and circulating thyroid-stimulating autoantibodies were negative in all but 1 tested patient [6]. Emotional disturbances and hyperkinetic behavior are very frequent in patients with PRTH, but both are also present in two-thirds of patients with GRTH (table 1). These findings show that there is a considerable overlap of clinical signs and symptoms among patients with PRTH and those with GRTH. Moreover, we found that clinical features of PRTH may vary in the same subject from time to time (table 2), indicating that factors other than the resistance play a role in the clinical presentation of the disease and, therefore, that a diagnosis of PRTH may be mistakenly made. Interestingly, the only symptom that was always present was anxiety, whose low specificity as indicator of a hyperthyroid state is well known.

High concentrations of circulating thyroid hormones in the presence of detectable TSH levels characterize both PRTH and GRTH without significant differences between the two forms. It has to be stressed the importance of measuring with direct methods the free moiety of circulating thyroid hormones instead of the total one in order to prevent possible misinterpretation due to variation of thyroid hormone transport proteins. Moreover, the use of free thyroid hormone measurement methods based on the 'analog' technique should be avoided, owing to the interference produced in such assays by both normal and abnormal serum transport proteins (familial dysalbuminemic hyperthyroxinemia, circulating anti-T_4 and/or anti-T_3 autoantibodies) [6, 22]. Contrary to previous RIAs, the new immunometric assays for TSH measurement, based on the 'sandwich' technique between TSH molecules and anti-TSH monoclonal antibodies, appear devoid of possible interferences which gave spuriously high TSH levels in RIAs [6].

About one-fifth of patients with PRTH and one-third of those with GRTH show TSH levels lying in the normal range, and no correlation between free thyroid hormone and TSH levels was observed. The enhanced biological activity of secreted TSH molecules (see below) may account for this unexpected finding. In the majority of patients with either PRTH or GRTH, the levels of circulating free α-SU, as well as α-SU/TSH molar ratio, are in the normal range. Although previous studies have suggested that an α-SU/TSH molar ratio below 1.0 is indicative of the presence of thyroid hormone resistance and rules out the presence of a TSH-secreting pituitary adenoma, the finding of α-SU/TSH molar ratios ranging from 5.5 to 29.1 in normal subjects indicates the need of comparing the individual values with those recorded in control groups matched for TSH and gonadotropin levels before any diagnostic conclusions are drawn [21].

Table 1. Clinical and biochemical characteristics of patients with PRTH as compared to those with GRTH

Feature	PRTH (n = 65)	GRTH (n = 260)
Age (range)	1.3–80	0.1–75
Sex (F:M)	45:20	141:119
Familial cases	32%	88%
Previous thyroid ablation	67%	57%
Goiter	93%	94%
Tachycardia	94%	80%
Emotional disturbances	88%	62%
Hyperkinetic behavior	88%	68%
Normal TSH levels	21%	32%
Normal α-SU levels	98%	99%
Normal α-SU/TSH mr	99%	98%

Measurement of Parameters of Peripheral Thyroid Hormone Action

As stated above, the finding of values compatible with hyperthyroidism of at least one parameter evaluating the peripheral thyroid hormone action, seems to be necessary for the diagnosis of PRTH. Therefore, the measurement of both in vivo (basal metabolic rate, cardiac systolic time intervals, Achilles tendon reflex time) and in vitro (SHBG, bone GLA protein, angiotensin-converting enzyme, soluble interleukin-2 receptor circulating in serum, blood red cell Na^+ content, etc.) parameters of peripheral thyroid hormone action is mandatory in the diagnostic procedure of resistant patients. However, the parameters to gauge thyroid hormone action in diverse tissues are limited and somewhat qualitative. Their clinical specificity and sensitivity are in general very low (<60%), with the exception of the measurement of SHBG whose specificity and sensitivity in indicating the absence or the presence of hyperthyroidism are 73 and 81%, respectively. We measured SHBG levels in 15 patients with PRTH and found that all had normal levels of this glycoprotein [9]. These data suggest that the resistance to thyroid hormone

Table 2. Spontaneous variations of some clinical signs and symptoms in 3 untreated patients with PRTH

Control	Pulse rate	Weight loss	Tremor	Asthenia	Anxiety	Increased sweating
Patient ADG						
First observation	96	+	–	+++	+++	++
After 5 months	64	–	++	–	++	–
Patient GP						
First observation	72	–	+	++	+++	+++
After 1 month	72	+	++	–	+	–
After 6 months	84	–	–	–	+	++
After 11 months	74	–	+	–	++	–
Patient MB						
First observation	98	+	++	++	+++	+
After 2 months	68	++	–	–	+++	–
After 8 months	96	–	–	++	+	+

in patients with PRTH is not selective at the pituitary level, but also involves liver cells. To further investigate this matter, we evaluated some parameters of peripheral thyroid hormone action in a series of 10 patients with PRTH and 20 with GRTH (table 3). The results confirm that, in a significant number of patients thought to be pituitary-resistant on a clinical ground, most parameters are in the normal range, thus indicating the presence of refractoriness to high thyroid hormone levels at the level of both pituitary and peripheral tissues. Indeed, bone GLA protein (osteocalcin) was normal in all tested patients with PRTH, thus indicating that the resistance in these subjects involves not only pituitary and hepatic tissues, but also the bones. On the contrary, due to the low specificity and sensitivity of such measurements, many patients with GRTH, i.e. without any clinical stigmata of peripheral hyperthyroidism, had values of some parameters of peripheral thyroid hormone action in the hyperthyroid range (table 3). Finally, in some patients with PRTH, the administration of T_3 at TSH-suppressive doses (100 µg/day/10 days) did not cause any increase in SHBG and bone GLA protein levels. Similar results have been previously reported by Sarne et al. [23] in patients with GRTH.

Table 3. Parameters of peripheral thyroid hormone action in patients with PRTH (n = 10) and GRTH (n = 20): percent of values in the hyperthyroid range (our series)

Form	PEP/LVET	SHBG nmol/l	BGP µg/l	ACE U/l	sIL-2R kU/l
PRTH	83	0	0	33	20
GRTH	60	14	20	62	40

PEP/LVET = Pre-ejection period/left ventricular ejection time; SHBG = sex hormone-binding globulin; BGP = bone GLA protein; ACE = angiotensin-converting enzyme; sIL-2R = soluble interleukin-2 receptor circulating in serum.

TSH Response to Dynamic Testing

Several stimulatory and inhibitory tests have been employed in order to evaluate TSH secretory dynamics in patients with PRTH and GRTH. In general, no significant differences between the two forms of resistance could be observed. TRH injection generally causes normal or even exaggerated and prolonged TSH responses [1–3, 24–30]. Dopamine antagonists, such as domperidone or sulpiride, cause TSH secretion to be normally increased in most patients with very few exceptions [31]. On the contrary, a normal response to T_3 suppression test, i.e. complete inhibition of TSH secretion both in basal conditions and after TRH stimulation, has never been recorded [23, 25].

Relationship between Structure and Function of Circulating TSH

To further investigate possible differences between PRTH and GRTH, we carried out experiments on the pattern of lectin binding as well as on bioactivity of circu-

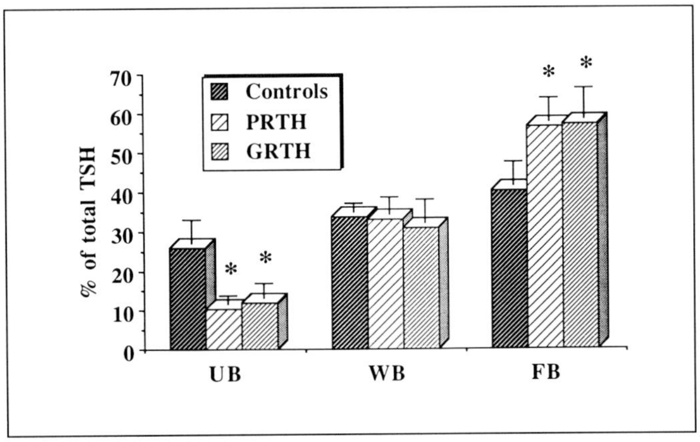

Fig. 2. Con A affinity chromatography of circulating TSH from normal controls and patients with PRTH and GRTH. Data (mean ± SD) are expressed as percent of total TSH added to Con A column. The unbound (UB) fraction contains molecules characterized by triantennary, tetra-antennary and bisecting oligosaccharide structures. The bound fractions were eluted with 10 m*M* α-methylglucopyranoside (weakly bound (WB) fraction containing molecules characterized by biantennary and truncated hybrid structures) followed by 300 m*M* α-methylmannopyranoside (firmly bound (FB) fraction containing molecules characterized by high mannose and hybrid structures). Fractions (1 ml) were collected and TSH measured by Delfia® in each fraction. * $p < 0.01$ vs. controls.

Table 4. Suggested modalities for PRTH treatment

Drug	Untoward effects and limitations
Antithyroid drugs	Further increase in TSH circulating levels: – Increase in goiter size – Risk for the development of TSH-secreting pituitary tumor (?)
Propranolol	Effects limited to β-adrenergic blockade and inhibition of peripheral T_4 to T_3 conversion
Corticosteroids	Cushingoid feature and inhibition of hypothalamic-pituitary-adrenal axis
Bromocriptine	Transient effects due to TSH escape from inhibition
Octreotide	Transient effects due to TSH escape from inhibition
L-T_3	Daily peaks of very high T_3 levels which maintain the hyperthyroid state
TRIAC	Effective in the majority of patients
D-T_4	Effective in the majority of patients

lating TSH. Lectins are proteins that specifically bind carbohydrate structures. Affinity chromatography of glycopeptides on immobilized lectins, such as concanavalin A (Con A), has been proven to be a powerful method for oligosaccharide fractionation [32]. N-linked oligosaccharide structures were shown to interact with Con A according to their branching properties as follows: triantennary, tetra-antennary and bisecting oligosaccharides do not bind to Con A, biantennary and truncated hybrids weakly bind to Con A, and high mannose and hybrid oligosaccharides firmly bind to Con A. As shown in figure 2, sera from resistant patients contained a greater proportion of TSH that firmly bound to Con A, indicating a shift from multiantennary and/or bisecting structures to hybrid and/or high mannose forms, i.e. to the secretion of less mature forms. Again, no differences were recorded in circulating TSH from patients with PRTH and from those with GRTH.

The bioactivity of circulating TSH was measured as cAMP accumulation in cultures of Chinese hamster ovary cells transfected with the recombinant human receptor of TSH [33]. Surprisingly, TSH from 2 patients with PRTH and 3 with GRTH showed an enhanced biological activity which caused the biological to immunological activity ratio (B/I) to be significantly increased in both PRTH and GRTH as compared to normal controls (B/I in PRTH: 3.2 ± 0.1 (mean ± SD); in GRTH: 3.6 v 0.2; in controls: 1.2 ± 0.6; $p < 0.01$).

Genetic Studies of T_3 Receptor

The recent discovery that the c-erbA proto-oncogene encodes for thyroid hormone receptors (TR) has opened a new era in the studies of thyroid hormone resistance [13, 15–19]. It was demonstrated that GRTH is tightly linked to c-erbAβ gene [10] and, soon after, that diverse mutations in T_3-binding domain of $TR\beta_1$ receptor were present [11, 12, 15–17]. These mutations alter thyroid hormone binding to the receptor, thus resulting in the clinical appearance of the disease. Moreover, it has been shown that resistance occurs in patients with heterozygous mutations, since the mutant receptor inhibits the activity of the normal β- and α-receptors [14–16]. At present, only 1 patient with clinical evidence of PRTH has been studied and a single-point mutation was identified altering an arginine to histidine in codon 311 (R311H) [15]. In our series, genetic studies were carried out in 2 patients with familial PRTH by amplification and sequence of exons encoding $TR\beta_1$ and point mutations in the T_3-binding domain of the receptor (R315H and R315L) were found [Chatterjee et al., in preparation]. These mutations are similar to those previously recorded in 2 unrelated patients with GRTH [15]. It is possible, however, that the pituitary resistance in PRTH patients is secondary to a $TR\alpha_1$ mutation or a mutation in NH_2-terminus in $TR\beta_1$ or $TR\beta_2$, the latter being expressed only in the pituitary cells [34]. Nevertheless, even molecular biology studies failed to demonstrate clear differences between PRTH and GRTH.

Treatment

Difficulties similar to those recorded in the diagnostic procedures are also found in the treatment of PRTH. Although many different agents have been suggested for the treatment of this particular form of hyperthyroidism (table 4), the major goal of the therapy is to block pituitary secretion of TSH with drug deprived of thyromimetic effects on peripheral tissues in order to reduce the endogenous thyroid hormone secretion and, thus, the peripheral hyperthyroidism [6, 24–30]. Among them, two different thyroid hormone analogs, i.e. TRIAC [24, 27] and *D*-T_4 [29, 30], have been documented to be useful in causing TSH blockade with consequent restoration of an apparent euthyroid state, though lack of clinical benefits has been recorded in few cases [6, 28]. Periodic interruption of the treatment with these agents is recommended in order to re-examine the clinical status of the patient. However, attention has to be paid to possible misdiagnosis of PRTH, as the above drugs are potentially dangerous in patients with GRTH whose compensated hypothyroidism may worsen.

Conclusions

Taken together, the above findings indicate that the existence of pituitary resistance to thyroid hormones as a definite clinical entity, clearly separated from GRTH, is questionable. On the contrary, they support the view that the various forms of thyroid hormone resistance may be part of a spectrum of disease with variable expression in different tissues. To better understand the variable clinical features that result from thyroid hormone resistance it will be necessary to acquire more information about the in vivo distribution, tissue specificity, regulation and mechanisms of action of both normal and mutant thyroid hormone receptors.

Acknowledgments

The authors are particularly indebted to Dr. V.K.K. Chatterjee (Cambridge, UK), who performed the genetic studies reported in the present paper, for the invaluable help and the fruitful discussion in the preparation of the manuscript.

This work was partially supported by grants from Murst and CNR (Rome, Italy) and Ospedale Maggiore IRCCS (Milan, Italy).

References

1 Refetoff S: Syndromes of thyroid hormone resistance. Am J Physiol 1982;43:E88–98.
2 Refetoff S, Salazar A, Smith TJ, Scherberg NH: The consequences of inappropriate treatment because of failure to recognize the syndrome of pituitary and peripheral tissue resistance to thyroid hormone. Metabolism 1983;32:822–833.
3 Refetoff S: Resistance to thyroid hormone revisited; in Oppenheimer JH (ed): Thyroid Today. 1–11, 1990, vol XIII, No 3.
4 Gershengorn MC, Weintraub BD: Thyrotropin-induced hyperthyroidism caused by selective pituitary resistance to thyroid hormone. A new syndrome of inappropriate secretion of TSH. J Clin Invest 1975;56:633–642.
5 Weintraub BD, Gershengorn MC, Kourides IA, Fein H: Inappropriate secretion of thyroid-stimulating hormone. Ann Intern Med 1981;95:339–351.
6 Faglia G, Beck-Peccoz P, Piscitelli G, Medri G: Inappropriate secretion of thyrotropin by the pituitary. Hormone Res 1987;26:79–99.
7 Complete list of references can be obtained from the authors.
8 Pagliara AS, Caplan RH, Gundersen CB, Wickhus GG, Elston AVC: Peripheral resistance to thyroid hormone in a family: Heterogeneity of clinical presentation. J Pediatr 1983;103:228–234.
9 Beck-Peccoz P, Roncoroni R, Mariotti S, Medri G, Marcocci C, Brabant G, Forloni F, Pinchera A, Faglia G: Sex hormone-binding globulin measurement in patients with inappropriate secretion of thyrotropin (IST): Evidence against selective pituitary thyroid hormone resistance in nonneoplastic IST. J Clin Endocrinol Metab 1990;71:19–25.
10 Usala SJ, Bale AE, Gesundheit N, et al: Tight linkage between the syndrome of generalized thyroid hormone resistance and the human c-erbAβ gene. Mol Endocrinol 1988;2:1217–1220.
11 Sakurai A, Takeda K, Ain K, Ceccarelli P, Nakai A, Seino S, Refetoff S, DeGroot LJ: Generalized resistance to thyroid hormone associated with a mutation in the ligand-binding domain of the human thyroid hormone receptor β. Proc Natl Acad Sci USA 1989;86:8977–8981.
12 Usala SJ, Tennyson GE, Bale AE, Lash RW, Gesundheit N, Wondisford FE, Acilli D, Hauser P, Weintraub BD: A base mutation of the c-erbA-beta thyroid hormone receptor in a kindred with generalized thyroid hormone resistance. Molecular heterogeneity in two other kindreds. J Clin Invest 1990;85:93–100.

13 Lazar MA, Chin WW: Nuclear thyroid hormone receptors. J Clin Invest 1990;86:1777–1782.
14 Chatterjee VKK, Nagaya T, Madison LD, Datta S, Rentoumis A, Jameson JL: Thyroid hormone resistance syndrome. Inhibition of normal receptor function by mutant thyroid hormone receptors. J Clin Invest 1991;87:1977–1984.
15 Usala SJ: Molecular diagnosis and characterization of thyroid hormone resistance syndromes. Thyroid 1991;1:361–367.
16 Usala SJ, Weintraub BD: Thyroid hormone resistance syndromes. Trends Endocrinol Metab 1991;2:140–144.
17 Takeda K, Weiss RE, Refetoff S: Rapid localization of mutations in the thyroid hormone receptor-β gene by denaturing gradient gel electrophoresis in 18 families with thyroid hormone resistance. J Clin Endocrinol Metab 1992;74:712–719.
18 Jameson JL: Thyroid hormone resistance: Pathophysiology at the molecular level (Editorial). J Clin Endocrinol Metab 1992;74:708–711.
19 De Nayer P: Generalized resistance to thyroid hormones. Hormone Res 1992;38:57–61.
20 Beck-Peccoz P, Piscitelli G, Amr S, Ballabio M, Bassetti M, Giannattasio G, Spada A, Nissim M, Weintraub BD, Faglia G: Endocrine, biochemical and morphological studies of a pituitary adenoma-secreting growth hormone, thyrotropin (TSH) and α-subunit: Evidence for secretion of TSH with increased bioactivity. J Clin Endocrinol Metab 1986;62:704–711.
21 Beck-Peccoz P, Persani L, Faglia G: Glycoprotein hormone α-subunit in pituitary adenomas. Trends Endocrinol Metab 1992;3:41–45.
22 Crinò A, Borrelli P, Salvatori R, Cortelazzi D, Roncoroni R, Beck-Peccoz P: Anti-iodothyronine autoantibodies in a girl with hyperthyroidism due to pituitary resistance to thyroid hormones. J Endocrinol Invest 1992;15:113–120.
23 Sarne DH, Refetoff S, Rosenfield RL, Farriaux JP: Sex hormone-binding globulin in the diagnosis of peripheral tissue resistance to thyroid hormone: The value of changes after short-term triiodothyronine administration. J Clin Endocrinol Metab 1988;66:740–746.
24 Beck-Peccoz P, Piscitelli G, Cattaneo MG, Faglia G: Successful treatment of hyperthyroidism due to nonneoplastic pituitary TSH hypersecretion with 3,5,3′-triiodothyroacetic acid. J Endocrinol Invest 1983;6:217–223.
25 Spanheimer RG, Bar RS, Hayford JC: Hyperthyroidism caused by inappropriate thyrotropin hypersecretion: Studies in patients with selective pituitary resistance to thyroid hormone. Arch Intern Med 1982;142:1283–1289.
26 Rösler A, Litvin Y, Hage C, Gross J, Cerasi E: Familial hyperthyroidism due to inappropriate thyrotropin secretion successfully treated with triiodothyronine. J Clin Endocrinol Metab 1982;54:76–82.
27 Salmela PI, Wide L, Juustila H, Ruokonen A: Effects of thyroid hormones (T_4, T_3), bromocriptine and TRIAC on inappropriate TSH hypersecretion. Clin Endocrinol (Oxf) 1988;28:497–507.
28 Kunitake JM, Hartman N, Henson LC, Lieberman J, Williams DE, Wong M, Hershman JM: 3,5,3′-Triiodothyroacetic acid therapy for thyroid hormone resistance. J Clin Endocrinol Metab 1989;69:46–52.
29 Hamon P, Bovier-Lapierre M, Robert M, Peynaud D, Pugeat M, Orgiazzi J: Hyperthyroidism due to selective pituitary resistance to thyroid hormones in a 15-month-old boy: efficacy of *D*-thyroxine therapy. J Clin Endocrinol Metab 1988;67:1089–1093.
30 Dorey F, Strauch G, Gayno JP: Thyrotoxicosis due to pituitary resistance to thyroid hormones. Successful control with *D*-thyroxine; a study in three patients. Clin Endocrinol (Oxf) 1990;32:221–227.
31 Benvenga S, Sobbrio GA, Vermiglio F, Li Calzi L, Cannavò S, Consolo F, Trimarchi F: Abnormal daily periodicity of serum thyrotropin (TSH) and evidence for defective TSH suppression in a case of non-neoplastic syndrome of inappropriate TSH secretion. J Endocrinol Invest 1987;10:195–202.
32 Papandréou MJ, Ronin C, Beck-Peccoz P: Oligosaccharide heterogeneity of human serum TSH in different clinical conditions as studied by concanavalin-A lectin-affinity chromatography. Thyroid 1991, 1(suppl 1):S86.
33 Persani L, Tonacchera M, Faglia G: Evaluation of circulating TSH bioactivity by means of cAMP accumulation in CHO cells transfected with recombinant human thyroid receptor of TSH (abstract). J Endocrinol Invest 1992; 15(suppl 2):4.
34 Hodin RA, Lazar MA, Wintman BI, Darling DS, Koenig RJ, Larsen PR, Moore DD, Chin WW: Identification of a thyroid hormone receptor that is pituitary-specific. Science 1989; 244:76–81.

Horm Res 1992;38:73–77

C. Toulas
P. Barraillé
F. Delassus
F. Bayard
H. Prats
J.-Ch. Faye

Institut L.-Bugnard, Laboratoire d'Endocrinologie Expérimentale INSERM CJF 9103, CHU Rangueil, Toulouse, France

Differential Initiation of Translation of a Single Estrogen Receptor mRNA Could Explain Some Estradiol Resistance Cases

Key Words
Steroid receptors
Resistance
Translation

Abstract
Cell response to steroid stimulation is generally acknowledged to be mediated by an intracellular protein known as a receptor. Response intensity is related to the affinity of the receptor and to the number of sites occupied by its specific ligand. Although verified in the majority of experimental and clinical studies, certain phenomena of steroid hormone resistance would seem to challenge this assertion. Application of gene molecular biology to determine the action mechanisms of steroid hormones has partially explained cell resistance in terms of genetic modifications. The work presented here shows that in certain cases, estrogen resistance could be explained by regulation of translation of the single messenger RNA coding for the receptor.

Introduction

By binding to their specific receptors, steroid hormones are able to influence gene expression in a wide variety of developmental and physiological processes in organisms as diverse as fungi and humans. The steroid receptors transduce extracellular hormonal signals to target genes that contain specific enhancer sequences referred to as hormone response elements. These receptors participate in a superfamily of gene expression regulatory proteins named transactivators. Comparative analysis of estrogen, progesterone and glucocorticoid receptors has revealed a typical structural organization in six homologous domains (A–F) [1] which has been extended to other members of the receptor superfamily [2]. Three major domains of activities were first identified in these proteins: (1) the hormone-binding domain in the carboxy-terminal region; (2) the DNA-binding domain in the medium region, and (3) two transactivating domains located in the NH_2-terminus and at the level of the hormone-binding domain [3]. A mutation in any one of these receptor domains might induce steroid cell resistance for all the target genes, and a mutation in the hormone-responsive element could also provoke this phenomenon but only for the proximal target gene.

These mutational events may be connected with the three major steroid-resistant phenotypes described by Sibley and Tomkins [4] whose work for a long time lead

J.-Ch. Faye
Institut L.-Bugnard
Laboratoire d'Endocrinologie Expérimentale
INSERM CJF 9103, CHU Rangueil
F–31054 Toulouse (France)

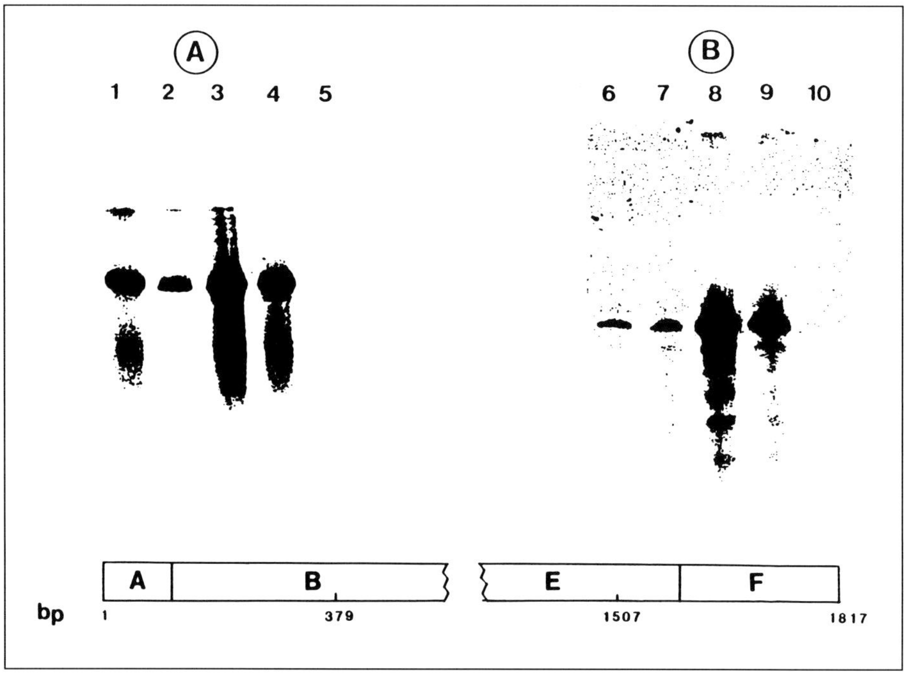

Fig. 1. ER gene transcription of MCF-7 cells in sensitive and refractory state. 10 μg of total RNA were analyzed using the RNase protection assay. ^{32}P-labeled antisense mRNA fragments were hybridized with ER mRNA and protected against RNaseA degradation. The protected bands were separated on 6% PAGE gels and were visualized by autoradiography. **A** Lanes 1–5: riboprobe of A/B domains (bp+1 to +379). **B** Lanes 6–10: riboprobe of E/F domains (bp +1507 to +1817). Negative controls with HeLa RNA (lanes 5, 10). MCF-7 cells: in estrogen-sensitive state (lanes 1, 6); in estrogen-sensitive state, grown in presence of E_2 (10^{-8} *M*) for 3 days (lanes 3, 8); in estrogen refractory state, grown in presence of E_2 (10^{-8} *M*) for 3 days (lanes 4, 9).

research on receptor steroid structure heterogeneity. In the case of the estrogen receptor (ER), many reports have related the presence of various polypeptidic structures in breast cancer tissues. The definition of their origins and the significance of such different receptor forms have sustained considerable debate [5–7]. However, until the application of gene molecular biology, no study had been able to completely exclude an unspecific proteolysis of the receptor [8, 12–13]. Although these tools have recently shown, in breast tumors, that some estrogen resistance could be associated with variant receptor mRNA [9, 10], the paradoxical ability of injected estrogen initially to stimulate and subsequently to inhibit the responsiveness of the uterus to further estrogen treatment observed by Stormshak et al. [11] cannot be explained by a mutation in the receptor gene since this effect is reversible and is observed in physiology [6]. This phenomenon was also observed in vitro on the breast cancer cell line MCF-7 [7] where cell estrogen sensitiveness was positively correlated with ER protein structure. We had shown in these reports that a 67-kD protein corresponds to the estrogen-sensitive state whereas a 45-kD protein was representative of the 'refractory state', both receptor forms were able to bind estrogen with the same affinity.

Using the radiation target theory [14] we have previously shown that ER bound to an antiestrogen was, in the whole cell, part of a 265-kD polypeptide structure if measured in estrogen-sensible cells or of 360-kD species in estrogen 'refractory' cells [15]. This work, which does not explain the origin of receptor heterogeneity, confirms that the size of the multimeric complex containing ER varies with cell estrogen sensitiveness.

Transcriptional Regulation of ER mRNA in MCF-7 Cells

Variant ER mRNA species detected in the trout liver [16] and in human cancer [10, 17] led it to be thought that the different forms of ER originated from transcriptional regulation of the gene. Moreover, other members of the superfamily are submitted to this regulation: multiple isoforms of both mouse retinoic acid receptors [18, 19] and chicken progesterone receptor [20] are generated by alternative splicing. These mRNA isoforms generated by the same gene by differential promoter usage differ in their 5′ regions. In a way to investigate the possibility of an alternative splicing of the ER mRNA, a ^{32}P-labeled antisense RNA was used to map the mRNA corresponding to the ER-binding domain (E/F). This riboprobe would be stable in both cases whereas a probe mapping the transactivator domain (A/B) would, on the contrary, exhibit different hybridations depending on the estrogen responsiveness of the cell. Figure 1 shows that bands representing the fully

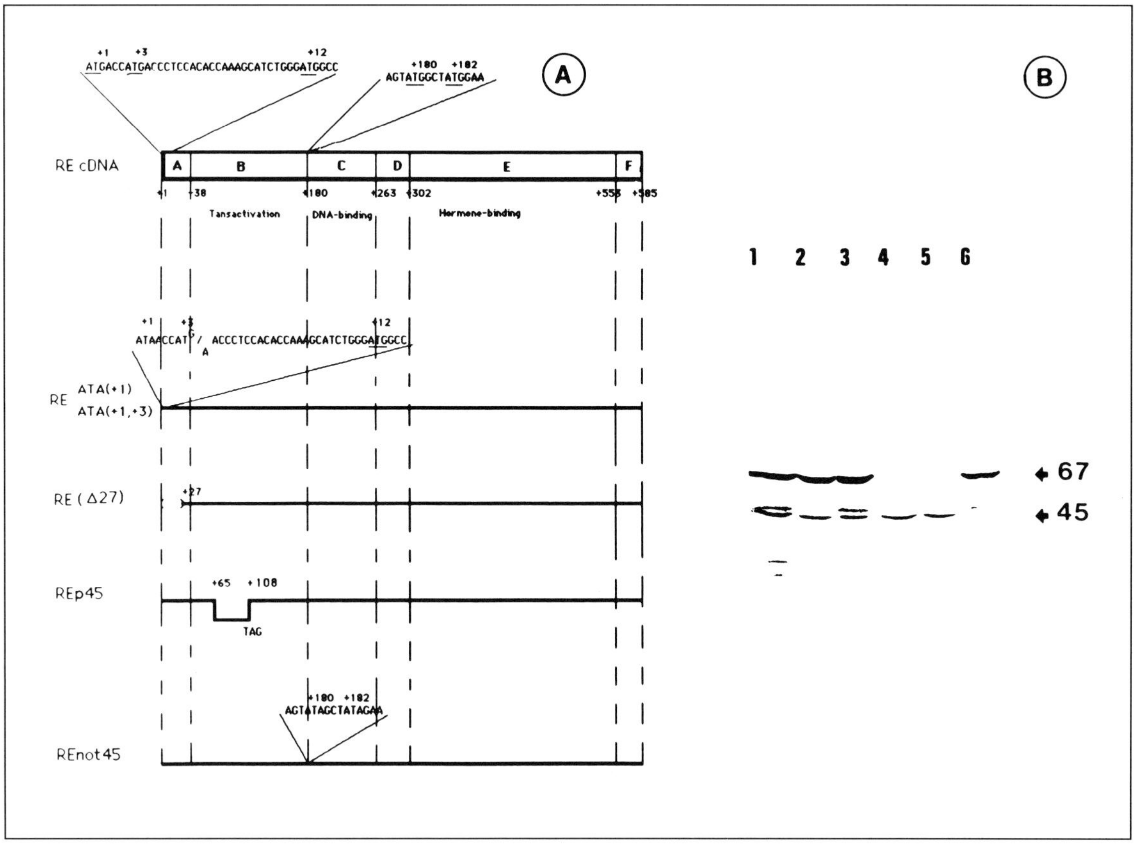

Fig. 2. A Human ER cDNA and constructed mutants. **B** Expression of ER and mutants in vitro. Autoradiographic analysis of polypeptides expressed from: the complete open reading frame cDNA (lane 1); mutated ER ATA+1 (lane 2); ER ATA+1 and ATA+3 (lane 3); deleted ER (Δ27) (lane 4); mutated ERp45 (lane 5); mutated ERnot45 (lane 6).

protected RNA fragments after RNase digestion were identical, whatever the state of the cell, with the two riboprobes (lanes 1–4, probe E/F; lanes 8–11, probe A/B); estradiol (10^{-8} *M*) has no effect on the protection (lanes 2, 4, 9, 11). We conclude that the human ER does not exhibit, by RNase mapping studies, different mRNA as the source of its sensitive (67-kD) and insensitive (45-kD) forms.

Alternate Initiation of Translation of a Unique mRNA Could Explain the Two Major Forms (67 and 45 kD) of ER

Analysis of the nucleotidic sequence of the cDNA encoding ER has led to the observation that over the first translation initiator ATG, other codons into the open reading frame are in a good nucleotidic context to initiate translation [21]. We therefore investigated by deletions and directed mutagenesis, the alternative initiations of translation of the ER mRNA as a possible control of the different protein forms (fig. 2).

The 1.8-kb cDNA fragment which contains the complete ER open reading frame provided by Prof. Chambon and the derived mutants (fig. 2A) were insert in the PSG5 vector such that large amounts of ER mRNA could be produced in vitro using T7 polymerase. ^{35}S-methionine was incorporated by in vitro translation using a rabbit reticulocyte lysate system and permitted the determination of the size of the mutant proteins (fig. 2B). As shown in figure 2B (lane 1) the complete ER mRNA gave rise to several products of which the 67- and 45-kD forms were the most expressed. Mutations of the AUG codons No. 1 and/or 3 in ATA led no unexpectedly similar profiles (lanes 2, 3) which could be explained by an initiation at AUG +12. Deletion of the 5′ region up to codon +27

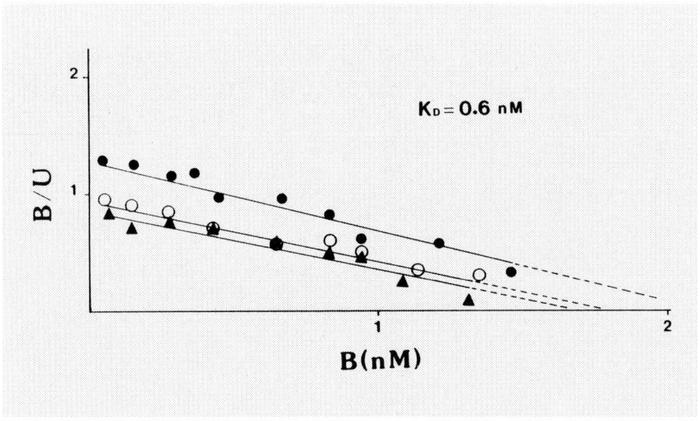

Fig. 3. Scatchard analysis of ER and mutants expressed in vivo. ERcDNA (●), ERp45 (▲), and ERnot45 (○) were transitorily expressed in Cos-7 cells and binding study was performed as previously described [6].

induced the disappearance of the 67-kD product without affecting expression of the 45-kD form (lane 4). Mutation on the codon +65 involving a change in the open reading frame and a AUG stop codon at +108 produced the same result (lane 5). Finally, change of both AUG +180 and +182 in ATA induced disappearance of the 45-kD product (lane 6).

Similar studies involving transitory transfections of different cDNA into COS-7 cells gave the same results (data not given) and showed that the proteins produced by ERp45 and ERnot45 plasmids were able to bind estradiol with the same affinity as cDNA possessing the entire open reading frame (fig. 3). These observations support the hypothesis that different initiations of the ER mRNA translation are partly accountable for the ER heterogeneity.

Conclusion

Steroid hormone activity via specific receptors is modulated by different cellular mechanisms as has been demonstrated by gene molecular biology. Genetic mutations of genes coding for hormone receptor proteins, in different domains, often induce different cell responses to the hormone under consideration. At the level of gene transcription in this family of receptors, alternative splicing of the RNA was shown to be responsible for certain heterogeneities in the peptide structure of progesterone receptors [20] and retinoic acid receptors [18, 19]. Within the limits of current knowledge, it would seem that each observation of a given receptor may also be found on another receptor in the superfamily. We show here that ER heterogeneity may be partly explained by regulation of the translation of a single messenger RNA. This mechanism would have the advantage of explaining certain paradoxes of estrogenic activity demonstrated in different tissues and cell lines [4, 7, 11].

Acknowledgements

This work was supported by the INSERM, the Association pour la Recherche contre le Cancer, and the Conseil Régional de Midi-Pyrénées. We thank Prof. Chambon for the generous gift of the cDNA for ER.

References

1 Kumar V, Green S, Stack G, Berry M, Jin JR, Chambon P: Functional domains of the human estrogen receptor. Cell 1987;51:941–951.
2 Wahli W, Martinez E: Superfamily of steroid nuclear receptors: Positive and negative regulators of gene expression. FASEB J 1991;5:2243–2249.
3 Kumar V, Green S, Staub A, Chambon P: Localisation of the oestradiol-binding and putative DNA-binding domains of the human oestrogen receptor. EMBO J 1986;5:2231–2236.
4 Sibley CH, Tomkins GM: Mechanisms of steroid resistance. Cell 1974;2:221–227.
5 Wiehle RD, Wittliff JL: Isoforms of estrogen receptors by high-performance ion-exchange chromatography. J Chromatogr 1984;197:313–326.
6 Faye J-Ch, Fargin A, Bayard F: Dissimilarities between the uterine estrogen receptor cytosol of castrated and estradiol-treated rats. Endocrinology 1986;118:2276–2283.
7 Faye J-Ch, Toulas C, Bayard F: Differential estrogenic responsiveness of MCF-7 cells: Relationship to the presence of two different estrogen receptors. J Recept Res 1989;9:203–219.
8 Sherman MR, Moran MC, Tuazon FB, Stevens YW: Structure, dissociation, and proteolysis of mammalian steroid receptors. J Biol Chem 1983;258:10366–10377.
9 Scott GK, Kushner P, Vigne JL, Benz CC: Truncated forms of DNA-binding estrogen receptors in human breast cancer. J Clin Invest 1991;88:700–706.
10 Murphy LC, Dotzlaw H: Variant estrogen receptor mRNA species detected in human breast cancer biopsy samples. Mol Endocrinol 1989;3:687–693.

11 Stormshak F, Leake R, Wertz N, Gorski J: Stimulatory and inhibitory effects of estrogen on uterine DNA systhesis. Endocrinology 1976;99:1501–1511.

12 Baskevitch PP, Rochefort H: A cytosol protease from the estrogen-resistant C3H mammary carcinoma increases the affinity of the estrogen receptor for DNA in vitro. Eur J Biochem 1985;146:671–678.

13 Horigome T, Ogata F, Golding TS, Korach K: Estradiol-stimulated proteolytic cleavage of the estrogen receptor in mouse uterus. Endocrinology 1988;123:2540–2548.

14 Lea DE: Action of Radiations on Living Cells. Cambridge, Cambridge University Press, 1955, pp 69–99.

15 Toulas C, Beauregard G, Delassus F, Thauvette L, Potier M, Bayard F, Faye J-Ch: Target size of estrogen receptor in cultured intact cells: Change in receptor structure between subconfluency and superconfluency in culture. Mol Cell Endocrinol 1972;72:89–94.

16 Pakdel F, Le Guellec C, Vaillant C, Le Roux MG, Valotaire Y: Identification and estrogen induction of two estrogen recptor (ER) messenger ribonucleic acids in the rainbow trout liver: Sequence homology with other ERs. Mol Endocrinol 1989;3:44–51.

17 Yaich L, Dupont WD, Cavener DR, Parl FF: Analysis of the PvuII restriction fragment-length polymorphism and exon structure of the estrogen receptor gene in breast cancer and peripheral blood. Cancer Res 1992;52:77–83.

18 Leroy P, Krust A, Zelent A, Mendelsohn C, Garnier JM, Kastner P, Dierich A, Chambon P: Multiple isoforms of the mouse retinoic acid receptor are generated by alternative splicing and differential induction by retinoic acid. EMBO J 1991;10:59–69.

19 Zelent A, Mendelsohn C, Kastner P, Krust A, Garnier JM, Ruffenach F, Chambon P: Differentially expressed isoforms of the mouse retinoic acid receptor β are generated by usage of two promoters and alternative splicing. EMBO J 1991;10:71–81.

20 Jeltsch JM, Turcottes B, Garnier JM, Lerouge T, Krozowski Z, Gronemeyer H, Chambon P: Characterization of multiple mRNAs originating from the chicken progesterone receptor gene. J Biol Chem 1990;265:3967–3974.

21 Kozak M: Bifunctional messenger RNAs in eucaryotes. Cell 1986;47:481–483.

Horm Res 1992;38:78–83

L. Caccavelli[a]
D. Cussac[a]
I. Pellegrini[b]
V. Audinot[a]
P. Jaquet[b]
A. Enjalbert[a]

[a] U. 159 INSERM, Paris;
[b] U. 297 INSERM, UER Médecine Nord, Marseille, France

D_2 Dopaminergic Receptors: Normal and Abnormal Transduction Mechanisms

Key Words
D_2 dopamine receptors
G proteins
Prolactinomas
PLA_2
PLC

Abstract
Dopamine receptors of D_2 type present on lactotroph cells are coupled to a large series of transduction mechanisms. Beside their negative coupling with adenylate cyclase, they are also coupled with potassium and calcium channels, leading to a decreased intracellular calcium concentration. In addition, D_2 dopamine receptors also modulate phospholipase activities. Dopamine inhibits inositol phosphate production, through two distinct mechanisms. One of them could represent a direct negative coupling with phospholipase C. All these transduction mechanisms of the D_2 dopamine receptors implicate G proteins sensitive to pertussis toxin. In contrast, these receptors are negatively coupled to phospholipase A_2 through G proteins insensitive to this toxin. Both isoforms of the D_2 dopamine receptor, generated by alternate splicing of a single gene, are present in lactotroph cells. After transfection in CH_4C_1 cells the two isoforms are coupled with adenylate cyclase while only the shortest isoform appears negatively coupled to phospholipase C. Functional D_2 dopamine receptors are present in human prolactinomas. Resistance to bromocriptine therapy is associated with a decreased density of these receptors in the tumor. In addition, the ratio of the two receptor isoforms (measured by PCR) is different in responsive and resistant tumors. Furthermore, the activity of Gi/Go proteins coupled to adenylate cyclase appears also affected in resistant tumors. Resistance to bromocriptine therapy appears thus to involve multiple changes at the different levels of the multiple mechanisms of action of dopamine on lactotroph cells.

Introduction

Dopamine represents the major inhibitor of prolactin release. Dopamine agonists such as bromocriptine [1] or other ergot derivatives [2], and more recently CV205–502 [3] have been successfully used for the treatment of patients with prolactin-secreting tumors. However, such treatments have not invariably reduced prolactin secretion in prolactinoma patients and in some patients a further tumor growth occurs despite the therapy [4, 5].

A. Enjalbert
U 159 INSERM
Centre Paul-Broca
2ter, rue d'Alésia
F–75014 Paris (France)

0301–0163/92/0382–0078
$2.75/0

We will first summarize the mechanism of action of dopamine on lactotroph cells and then the possible impairments of these mechanisms which could account for the resistance to dopaminergic therapy of prolactinoma patients.

D_2 Dopamine Receptors and G Proteins

Dopamine inhibition of prolactin secretion is mediated by D_2 dopamine receptors expressed by lactotroph cells [6]. These receptors belong to the family of G protein-coupled receptors, which comprise a single polypeptide chain containing seven hydrophobic transmembrane domains. The transducing G proteins also belong to a large family of molecules, called GTPases for their property to bind and hydrolyze GTP. These proteins exist under two major steps, one active with GTP bound, another inactive when GDP is present. They play the role of a molecular switch in a large number of cellular functions [7]. G proteins involved in signal transduction are heterotrimers $\alpha\beta\gamma$. Membrane receptor activation by an agonist facilitates GTP binding by increasing release of GDP from α subunits. The activated form of G proteins will activate or inactivate a large number of effector systems such as enzymes (adenylate cyclase, phospholipase C, phospholipase A_2) or ionic channels (Ca^{2+} channels, K^+ channels ...) [8]. There are several α subunits which exhibit differential sensitivity towards GTP, Mg^{2+} and bacterial toxins (cholera toxin, *Bordetella pertussis* toxin).

D_2 Dopamine Receptors and cAMP

D_2 dopamine receptors in lactotroph cells are negatively coupled to adenylate cyclase [9–11]. This property initially allowed to distinguish these receptors from D_1 receptors which are positively coupled to the enzyme [12]. This negative coupling of D_2 dopamine receptors is mediated by Gi/Go proteins sensitive to pertussis toxin [13].

Several α subunits of G proteins are present in anterior pituitary cells, three of them, at least, being substrates of pertussis toxin [14], and corresponding to $\alpha i_{1\text{-}2}$, α_0 and αi_3 [15]. Purification studies indicate that D_2 receptors are associated with Go and Gi proteins [16]. Furthermore, direct activation of G proteins by D_2 dopamine receptors could be determined by binding of GTP analogues on membranes of anterior pituitary cells [15].

The same G protein does not seem to be implicated in the negative coupling of various neurohormone receptors with adenylate cyclase in lactotrophs. This is attested by the differential GTP sensitivity of adenylate cyclase inhibition by DA on one hand, and angiotensin II [17] or somatostatin [18] on the other hand.

This difference in the coupling mechanisms of dopamine and somatostatin receptors with adenylate cyclase is further substantiated by the differential effect of estradiol [19]. It is well established that steroid hormones modulate pituitary responsiveness towards neurohormones. Estradiol increases the number of somatostatin receptors, and this accounts for the increased responsiveness of adenylate cyclase and prolactin secretion. In contrast, estradiol selectively affects the coupling mechanism of the dopamine receptors, leading to a marked reduction of dopamine-induced inhibition of adenylate cyclase activity without affecting the dopaminergic binding sites [20].

The steroid also induced a marked increase of protein kinase C activity, both in the cytosol and the membranes of anterior pituitary cells [21] which could contribute to the steroid effect on the cell sensitivity.

D_2 Dopaminergic Receptors and Calcium

D_2 dopamine receptors, beside their effect on adenylate cyclase, are able to inhibit inositol phosphate production [22–24]. This effect also involves G proteins sensitive to pertussis toxin [14]. The dopamine inhibition of inositol phosphate accumulation can be resolved into two distinct components [25]. One of them is the blockade of L type calcium channels. This is in agreement with the effect of dopamine on dihydropyridine agonist-induced prolactin secretion [26] on Ca^{2+} fluxes [27] as well as intracellular calcium concentrations [28].

In fact, dopamine has an effect on multiple Ca^{2+} and K^+ channels in lactotroph cells [29–31]. Interestingly, it seems that distinct G proteins are involved in the coupling of D_2 dopamine receptors with Ca^{2+} and K^+ channels. Go seems to be involved in the effects on Ca^{2+} currents, whereas Gi_3 could be implicated in the effect on K^+ currents [32].

Dihydropyridine antagonists, specific of L type calcium channels, partially mimic the dopamine effect on inositol phosphate production. Furthermore, the effects of the dihydropyridine and of dopamine are not additive. The second component of dopamine inhibition of inositol phosphate production is faster than the other one. Indeed, it can be demonstrated after 10 s incubation. This component of dopamine inhibition cannot be blocked by increasing intracellular Ca^{2+} concentrations induced by ionophores whereas these treatments completely suppressed the dihydropyridine inhibition [25].

These results are compatible with a negative coupling of D_2 dopamine receptors with phospholipase C, mediated by a G protein sensitive to pertussis toxin. Inhibition of phospholipase C by G proteins has been described in cerebral cortex membranes [33]. Other inhibitions of inositol phosphate production have been described, including the inhibition by adenosine (A1) of TRH-stimulated inositol phosphate production in GH_3 cells [34].

D_2 Dopamine Receptors and Arachidonic Acid

An additional effect of dopamine, inhibition of arachidonic acid release from pituitary cells, has also been recently reported [35 – 37].

This effect appears independent of the other transduction mechanisms of D_2 dopamine receptors that we have described so far [38]. It can be detected under basal conditions as well as after stimulation with TRH or angiotensin II. This dopamine inhibition is not affected by a 10-fold stimulation of cAMP levels by forskolin, and is still observed in the presence of high doses of A23187, a calcium ionophore. Furthermore, in contrast to the inhibition of inositol phosphate, this dopamine effect on arachidonic acid release is not inhibited by dihydropyridine antagonists. It is also unaffected by desensitization of protein kinase C by a long-term treatment with phorbol esters.

Finally, this dopamine inhibition has also been observed on membrane preparations, even after blockade of phospholipase C activity by neomycin [38]. This strongly suggests that D_2 dopamine receptors exhibit a direct, negative coupling with phospholipase A_2. G protein-dependent stimulation of phospholipase A_2 by GTP analogues has been reported in various models [39]. In anterior pituitary cells dopamine inhibited GTP or GTPγS stimulated arachidonic acid release. However, the dopamine effect was not sensitive to pertussis toxin, in contrast to all the other transduction mechanisms of D_2 dopamine receptors [38]. The coupling of D_2 receptors with phospholipase A_2 is thus likely to involve, at least partially, a non-PTX-sensitive G protein subunit. The latter mechanism could account for the pertussis toxin-unsensitive component of dopamine inhibition of prolactin secretion [40].

D_2 Dopamine Receptor Isoforms

D_2 dopamine receptors have been cloned [41]. They exist under two isoforms generated by alternative splicing [42]. Interestingly, both isoforms only differ by a 29 amino acid additive sequence located within the third intracytoplasmic loop known to interact with G proteins [43, 44]. Normal pituitary cells express both receptor isoforms [42, 45]. In contrast, GH_4C_1, a cell line which synthesizes and releases prolactin, is devoid of D_2 dopamine receptors [46]. These cells are thus the ideal model to transfect cDNA of D_2 dopamine receptors. We separately transfected each receptor isoform and established stable cell lines. In both cases, D_2 dopamine receptors are expressed by the cells, as attested by the presence of high affinity binding sites using iodosulpiride as ligand [47]. These receptors appear functional since they both mediate dopamine inhibition of prolactin secretion. In addition, dopamine inhibition of adenylate cyclase activity is observed with both isoforms. In contrast, inhibition of phospholipase C is observed only in GH_4C_1 cells transfected with the short receptor isoform. These results demonstrate the physiological importance of the third intracytoplasmic domain of the receptor in interacting with G proteins. They also indicate that distinct G proteins sensitive to pertussis toxin are coupled to adenylate cyclase on the one hand and phospholipase C on the other [47].

Resistance to Bromocriptine

Such a differential coupling of the two isoforms of D_2 dopamine receptors could imply functional differences in dopamine responses of different tissues containing variable proportions of these isoforms.

This functional difference of the two isoforms could also explain the fact that regulation of dopamine sensitivity, for example after long-term treatment with dopaminergic drugs, implies modulation of alternative splicing of the D_2 dopaminergic receptor gene both in brain [48] and pituitary [49].

The percentage of patients resistant to bromocriptine varies from 5 to 18% in different series. These patients are indistinguishable from bromocriptine-sensitive prolactinoma patients [50]. The resistant patients' adenomatous lactotrophs are relatively insensitive to the inhibitory effects of bromocriptine on prolactin secretion in vitro [50]. These resistant prolactinoma cells respond in the same way as do the tumor cells from responsive patients to other stimulatory or inhibitory neurohormones. These data thus support the hypothesis that the resistant cells have an isolated defect of their dopaminergic regulatory mechanisms. In fact, the density of dopaminergic binding sites is lower in resistant than in responsive tumors [50]. Furthermore, there is a good correlation between the density of D_2 dopaminergic binding sites and maximal dopamine inhibition of adenylate cyclase inhibition in the responsive adenomas as well as most of resistant adenomas, suggesting that the dopamine receptors present have the same type of coupling, quantitatively and qualitatively, to adenylate cyclase in these prolactinomas. Thus, the number of D_2 dopaminergic binding sites could be the limiting step of dopamine regulation in the resistant tumors.

It should be noted that in GH_3 cells, a tumoral cell line secreting prolactin, the defect of dopaminergic regulation of prolactin secretion can be accounted for by the absence of D_2 dopaminergic binding sites [46]. In this cell line, induction of such binding sites by growth factor treatment leads to the restoration of a dopamine inhibition of prolactin secretion [51].

In addition to this quantitative modification of D_2 dopamine receptors, we have also recently observed a significant difference in the ratio of the mRNA coding for the two D_2 dopamine receptor isoforms between prolactinoma from normally responsive and resistant patients [52]. A defect in the D_2 receptor short isoform expression could contribute to resistance to bromocriptine. In fact, this isoform could inhibit prolactin secretion by several mechanisms, some of them being not affected by the other receptor isoform.

Finally, in some cases in which resistance to bromocriptine was associated with tumor growth during therapy, a paradoxical stimulation of adenylate cyclase by dopamine is present [50].

In addition to modification at the level of D_2 dopamine receptor, an impairment in the coupling mechanisms with effector systems could thus be involved in resistance to bromocriptine.

In fact, we have observed an impairment of the activity of inhibitory G proteins coupled to adenylate cyclase of resistant tumors. This phenomenon could be associated with a relative reduced expression to αo subunit of G proteins. Interestingly, such a deficiency in αo subunit has been described in experimental tumors presenting a defect in dopamine regulation of prolactin secretion [53]. Furthermore, mutations of Gs proteins have been proposed to be involved in tumorigenesis of some cases of acromegalic pituitary tumors [54].

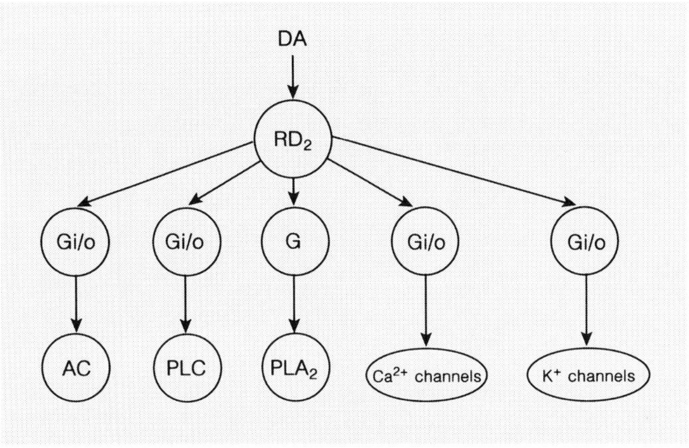

Fig. 1. Multiple transduction mechanisms of D_2 dopamine receptors in lactotrophs. DA = Dopamine; RD_2 = D_2 dopamine receptors; Gi/Go = G proteins, substrate of pertussis toxin; G = G protein unsensitive to pertussis toxin; AC = adenylate cyclase; PLC = phospholipase C; PLA_2 = phospholipase A_2; Ca^{2+} channels = voltage-sensitive calcium channels; K^+ channels = potassium channels.

Conclusion

D_2 dopamine receptor is a good example of membrane receptor coupled to G proteins which present several transduction mechanisms. In fact, these receptors appear able to inhibit most, it not all, the intracellular mechanisms involved in the regulation of prolactin release and synthesis (fig. 1).

These receptors interact with several members of the G protein family. Distinct G proteins seem to be involved in coupling with adenylate cyclase, phospholipase C, Ca^{2+} and K^+ channels and phospholipase A_2. Furthermore, isoforms of these receptors seem to present differential coupling mechanisms.

In prolactinomas, resistance to bromocriptine therapy also appears associated to more than one single modification. Quantitative modification of the expression of D_2 dopamine receptors, but perhaps also of G protein subunits, could be associated with qualitative changes in the ratio of D_2 dopamine receptor isoforms as well as in the activity of G proteins coupled to adenylate cyclase. Whether some of these defects can be accounted for by gene mutation in the regulatory sequences as well as in the sequences coding for these proteins remains to be determined.

References

1 Besser GM, Parkes L, Edwards CRW, Forsyth IA, McNeilly AS: Galactorrhea: Successful treatment with reduction of plasma prolactin levels by bromoergocryptine. BMJ 1972;iii: 669–672.

2 Crosignani PG, Ferrari C, Liuzzi A, Benco R, Mattei A, Rampini P, Dellabonzana D, Scarduelli C, Spelta B: Treatment of hyperprolactinemic states with different drugs: A study with bromocriptine, methoergoline and lisuride. Fertil Steril 1982;37(1):61–67.

3 Nordmann R, Petcher T: Octahydrobenzo-[g]quinoline: Potent dopamine agonists which show the relationship between ergolines and apomorphine. J Med Chem 1985;28:367–375.

4 Thorner MO, Besser GM: Bromocriptine treatment of hyperprolactinemic hypogonadism. Acta Endocrinol (Copenh) 1978;88(suppl): 131–146.

5 Werder KV, Fahlbusch R, Landgraf R, Pickardt CR, Rjosk HK, Scriba PC: Treatment of patients with prolactinomas. J Endocrinol Invest 1978;1:47–59.

6 Cronin MJ: The role and direct measurement of the dopamine receptor(s) in the anterior pituitary; in Muller EE, MacLeod RM (eds): Neuroendocrine Perspectives. Amsterdam, Elsevier, 1982, vol 1, pp 1–169.

7 Bourne HR, Sanders DA, McCormick F: The GTPase superfamily: A conserved switch for diverse cell functions. Nature 1990;348:125–132.

8 Birnbaumer L, Abramowitz J, Brown AM: Signal transduction of G proteins. Biochim Biophys Acta 1990;1031:163–224.

9 Giannattasio G, De Ferrari ME, Spada A: Dopamine-inhibited adenylate cyclase in female rat adenohypophysis. Life Sci 1981;28:1605–1611.

10 Enjalbert A, Bockaert J: Pharmacological characterization of the D_2 dopaminergic receptor negatively coupled with adenylate cyclase in rat anterior pituitary. Mol Pharmacol 1983;23: 576–584.

11 McDonald WH, Sibley DR, Kilpatrick BE, Caron MG: Dopaminergic inhibition of adenylate cyclase correlates with high affinity agonist binding to anterior pituitary D_2 dopamine receptors. Mol Cell Endocrinol 1984;36:201–209.

12 Kebabian JW, Calne DB: Multiple receptors for dopamine. Nature 1987;277:93–96.

13 Cronin MJ, Myers G, MacLeod RM, Hewlett EL: Pertussis toxin uncouples dopamine agonist inhibition of prolactin release. Am J Physiol 1983;244:E449–504.

14 Journot L, Homburger V, Pantaloni C, Priam M, Bockaert J, Enjalbert A: An islet activating protein sensitive G protein is involved in dopamine inhibition of angiotensin and thyrotropin releasing hormone stimulated inositol phosphate production in anterior pituitary cells. J Biol Chem 262:15106–15110.

15 Cussac D, Kordon C, Enjalbert A, Saltarelli S: VIP induced cross talk between G proteins in membranes from anterior pituitary cells. Cell Signal, 1993, in press.

16 Senogles SE, Benovic JL, Amlaiky N, Virson C, Milligan G, Vinistsky R, Spiegel AM, Caron MG: The D_2 dopamine receptor of anterior pituitary is functionally associated with a pertussis toxin sensitive gunanine nucleotide binding protein. J Biol Chem 1987;262:4860–4867.

17 Audinot V, Rasolonjanahary R, Bertrand P, Priam M, Kordon C, Enjalbert A: PKC modulation of inhibitory coupling of angiotensin II receptors with adenylate cyclase in lactotroph cells. Mol Cell Neurosci 1992;3:145–151.

18 Musset F, Bertrand P, Priam M, Kordon C, Enjalbert A: Differential coupling with pertussis toxin sensitive G proteins of dopamine and somatostatin receptors involved in regulation of adenohypophyseal secretion. Mol Cell Endocrinol 1990;73:1–10.

19 Enjalbert A, Bertrand P, Bockaert J, Drouva S, Kordon C: Multiple coupling of neurohormone receptors with cyclic AMP and inositol phosphate production in anterior pituitary cells. Biochimie 1987;69:271–279.

20 Maus M, Bertrand P, Drouva S, Rasolonjanahary R, Kordon C, Glowinski J, Prémont J, Enjalbert A: Differential effects of estradiol on D_1 and D_2 dopamine sensitive adenylate cyclase in anterior pituitary cells and striatal neurons in primary culture. J Neurochem 1989;52: 410–418.

21 Drouva SV, Gorenne I, Laplante E, Rérat E, Enjalbert A, Kordon C: Estradiol modulates protein kinase C activity in the rat pituitary in vivo and in vitro. Endocrinology 1990;126: 536–544.

22 Enjalbert A, Sladeczek F, Guillon G, Bertrand P, Shu C, Epelbaum J, Garcia-Sainz A, Jard S, Lombard C, Kordon C, Bockaert J: Angiotensin II and dopamine modulate both cAMP and inositol phosphate productions in anterior pituitary cells: Involvement in prolactin secretion. J Biol Chem 1986;26:4071–4075.

23 Vallar L, Vicentini LM, Meldolesi J: Inhibition of inositol phosphate production is a late Ca^{2+} dependent effect of D_2 dopaminergic receptor activation in rat lactotroph cells. J Biol Chem 1988;263:10127–10314.

24 Martinez de la Escalera G, Weiner RI: Effect of dopamine withdrawal on activation of adenylate cyclase and phospholipase C in enriched lactotroph cells. Endocrinology 1988;123: 1682–1687.

25 Enjalbert A, Guillon G, Mouillac B, Audinot V, Rasolonjanahary R, Kordon C, Bockaert J: Dual mechanism of inhibition by dopamine of basal and TRH stimulated inositol phosphate production in anterior pituitary cells. J Biol Chem 1990;265:18816–18822.

26 Enjalbert A, Musset F, Chénard C, Priam M, Kordon C, Heisler S: Dopamine inhibits prolactin secretion stimulated by the calcium channel agonist BAY-8644 through a pertussis toxin sensitive G protein in anterior pituitary cells. Endocrinology 1988;123:406–412.

27 Schofield JG: Use of a trapped fluorescent indicator to demonstrate effects of thyroliberin and dopamine on cytoplasmic calcium concentrations in bovine anterior pituitary cells. FEBS Lett 1983;159:79–82.

28 Malgaroli A, Vallar L, Elahi FR, Pozzan T, Spada A, Meldolesi J: Dopamine inhibits cytosolic Ca^{2+} increase in rat lactotroph cells. Evidence of a dual mechanism of action. J Biol Chem 1987;262:13920–13927.

29 Israel JM, Kirk C, Vincent JD: Electrophysiological responses to dopamine of rat hypophyseal cells in lactotroph enriched primary culture. J Physiol (Lond) 1987;390:1–22.

30 Lledo PM, Legendre P, Israel JM, Vincent JD: Dopamine inhibits two characterized voltage dependent calcium currents in identified rat lactotroph cells. Endocrinology 1990;127:990–1001.

31 Lledo PM, Legendre P, Zhang J, Israel JM, Vincent JD: Effects of dopamine on voltage dependent potassium currents on identified rat lactotroph cells. Neuroendocrinology 1990;52: 545–555.

32 Lledo PM, Homburger V, Bockaert J, Vincent JD: Differential G proteins and Ca^{++} currents in rat anterior pituitary cells. Neuron 1992;8: 455–463.

33 Litosch I: Guanine nucleotide mediates stimulatory and inhibitory effects on cerebral cortical membrane phospholipase C activity. Biochem J 1989;261:245–251.

34 Delahunty TM, Cronin M, Lunden J: Regulation of GH_3 cell function via adenosine A1 receptors. Inhibition of prolactin release, cyclic AMP production and inositol phosphate generation. Biochem J 1988;255:69–77.

35 Judd A, Ross PC, Spangelo BI, McLeod R: Angiotensin II increases pituitary cell prolactin release and arachidonate liberation. Mol Cell endocrinol 1988;57:115–121.

36 Canonico PL: D_2 dopamine receptor activation reduces free [^{3}H]-arachidonate release induced by hypophysiotropic peptides in anterior pituitary cells. Endocrinology 1989;125: 1180–1186.

37 Ohmichi M, Hirota K, Koike K, Kadowaki K, Yamaguchi M, Miyake A, Tanizawa O: Dopamine inhibits the arachidonate and prolactin release stimulated by thyrotropin-releasing hormone through an islet-activating protein sensitive GTP binding protein in anterior pituitary cells. Neuroendocrinology 1990;52:75–81.

38 Ponce G, Priam M, Gautron JP, Kordon C, Enjalbert A: Dopamine inhibition of arachidonic acid release is independent of other transduction mechanisms of D_2 dopamine receptors in anterior pituitary. Mol Cell Endocrinol, submitted.

39 Watkins DC, Northup JK, Malbon CC: Pertussis toxin treatment in vivo is associated with a decline in G-protein β-subunits. J Biol Chem 1989;264:4186–4194.
40 Musset M, Bertrand P, Priam M, Kordon C, Enjalbert A: Differential mechanisms of dopamine and somatostatin inhibition of prolactin secretion from anterior pituitary cells. J Neuroendocrinol 1991;3:21–28.
41 Bunzow JR, Van Tol HHM, Grandy DK, Albert PL, Salon J, Christie MC, Machida CA, Weve KA, Civelli O: Cloning and expression of a rat dopamine D_2 receptor cDNA. Nature 1988;336:783–787.
42 Giros B, Sokoloff P, Martres MP, Riou JF, Emorine L, Schwartz JC: Alternative splicing directs the expression of two D_2 dopamine receptor isoforms. Nature 1989;342:923–926.
43 Strader CD, Sigal IS, Dixon RAF: Structural basis of β-adrenergic receptor function. FASEB J 1989;3:1825–1832.
44 Cotecchia S, Exum S, Caron MG, Lefkowitz RJ: Regions of the α_1-adrenergic receptor involved in coupling to phosphatidylinositol hydrolysis and enhanced sensitivity of biological function. Proc Natl Acad Sci USA 1990;87: 2896–2900.
45 Dal Toso R, Sommer B, Ewert M, Herb A, Pritchell DB, Bach A, Smivers BD, Seeburg PH: The dopamine D_2 receptor: Two molecular forms generated by alternative splicing. EMBO J 1989;8:4025–4034.
46 Cronin MJ, Faure W, Martial J, Weiner RI: Absence of high affinity dopamine receptors in GH_3 cells: A prolactin secreting clone resistant to the inhibitory action of dopamine. Endocrinology 1980;106:718–723.
47 Audinot V, Rasolonjanahary R, Giros B, Martres MP, Sokoloff P, Schwartz JC, Kordon C, Enjalbert A: Couplage différentiel à la phospholipase C des deux isoformes du récepteur dopaminergique D_2 transfectées dans la ligne GH_4C_1. Ann Endocrinol 1991;52:17N.
48 Martres MP, Sokoloff P, Giros B, Schwartz JC: Effects of dopaminergic transmission interruption on the D_2 receptor isoforms in various cerebral tissues. J Neurochem 1992;58:673–679.
49 Arnaud E, Arsaut J, Demotes-Mainard J: Differential plasticity of the dopamine D_2 receptor mRNA isoforms, under haloperidol treatment, as evidenced by in situ hybridization in rat anterior pituitary. Neurosci Lett 1991;130:12–16.
50 Pellegrini I, Rasolonjanahary R, Gunz G, Bertrand P, Delivet S, Jedynak GP, Kordon C, Peillon F, Jaquet P, Enjalbert A: Resistance to bromocriptine in prolactinomas. J Clin Endocrinol Metab 1989;69:500–509.
51 Missale C, Castelletti L, Boroni F, Memo M, Spano P: Epidermal growth factor induces the functional expression of dopamine receptors in the GH3 cell line. Endocrinology 1991;127:13–20.
52 Chevalier L, Féron F, Morange I, Dewailly D, Jaquet P, Kordon C, Enjalbert A: Differential expression of two dopaminergic D_2 receptor isoforms in bromocriptine resistant prolactinomas. Abstracts of the 9th International Congress of Endocrinology, Nice 1992.
53 Bouvier C, Forget H, Lagacé G, Drews R, Sinnett D, Labuda D, Collu R: G proteins in normal rat pituitaries and in prolactin secreting rat pituitary tumors. Mol Cell Endocrinol 1991; 78:33–44.
54 Laundis C, Masters SR, Spada A, Pace AM, Bourne HR, Vallar L: GTPase inhibiting mutation activate the α chain of Gs and stimulate adenyl cyclase in human pituitary tumors. Nature 1989;340:692–696.

Horm Res 1992;38:84–89

T. Brue
I. Pellegrini
A. Priou
I. Morange
P. Jaquet

Service d'Endocrinologie et
Maladies Métaboliques, and
INSERM U. 297,
Centre Hospitalier Universitaire Nord,
Marseille, France

Prolactinomas and Resistance to Dopamine Agonists

Key Words
Prolactin-secreting adenoma
Pituitary adenoma
Bromocriptine
Resistance to bromocriptine
Dopamine agonists
CV 205-502

Abstract
Among 288 patients with prolactinoma (aged 12–62 years; 242 women), 27 were diagnosed as resistant to bromocriptine as their plasma prolactin (PRL) levels remained elevated despite long-term (3 months or more) treatment at high doses ($\geq$15 mg daily). These 18 women and 9 men, aged 29 $\pm$ 9 years (mean $\pm$ SD, range 13–50), followed-up for 8 $\pm$ 4 years, had microadenomas (n = 6) or macroadenomas. They were treated by dopamine agonists alone (n = 6) or associated with surgical or radiation therapy. In 8 cases repetitive surgical treatments were necessary. Among the 24 patients who were treated with the nonergot dopamine agonist CV 205-502 after unsuccessful bromocriptine treatment, half of them (9 women, 3 men) resumed normal PRL levels on doses ranging from 0.15 to 0.45 mg/day. Despite daily doses of CV 205-502 from 0.3 to 0.525 mg, the remaining patients were not normalized by this drug which did not prevent tumor growth in 4 of them. Two patients died from invasive cerebral extensions of their tumor and a third had vertebral metastases with positive anti-PRL immunostaining. It is concluded that bromocriptine-resistant prolactinomas represent the most severe aspect of this disease and that a more powerful dopamine agonist like CV 205-502 is effective in only a fraction of these patients.

Since it was introduced two decades ago [1] as an effective treatment of hyperprolactinemia, the prolactin (PRL) agonist bromocriptine has been extensively used in patients with PRL-secreting adenomas. Indeed, it is now well established that PRL secretion is under tonic inhibitory control by dopamine [2] and that both dopamine and its agonists are able to inhibit secretion from normal as well as adenomatous pituitary cells [3]. Many clinical studies have demonstrated that different dopamine agonists can induce both a drop in plasma PRL levels and a reduction in tumor size in most patients with PRL-secreting adenomas [4–7]. However, even when problems with compliance can be excluded using long-acting injectable bromocriptine preparations, a subset of patients with prolactinomas fail to respond to long-term bromocriptine treatment [8]. Moreover, earlier studies had shown the wide spectrum of sensitivity to bromocriptine in vivo since a single 2.5-mg oral dose was able to induce a 47-

Dr. T. Brue
Service d'Endocrinologie et Maladies Métaboliques
Centre Hospitalier Universitaire Nord
Chemin des Bourrelly
F–13015 Marseille (France)

0301–0163/92/0382–0084
$2.75/0

96% decrease in plasma PRL levels in hyperprolactinemic patients [9]. A fraction of the prolactinoma patients have thus been shown by several authors to be resistant to bromocriptine as such a treatment administered during 3 months or more at doses above 15 mg daily (i.e. at least twice the usually effective dose) failed to allow normalization of plasma PRL concentrations and a significant reduction in tumor size [4, 10–15].

In this paper we analyze our currently available clinical and biological data to try to address some questions raised by these dopamine-resistant prolactinomas.

Subjects and Methods

Among 383 patients (322 women; age range 13–63 years) treated in our center from 1976 to 1991 for PRL-secreting adenomas, 249 had macroadenomas (largest diameter >10 mm, basal PRL >200 mg/l) and 134 had microadenomas (tumor size <10 mm). Twenty-five percent of the whole population was treated by surgery only. In the remaining patients (n = 288), bromocriptine allowed normalization of plasma PRL levels in 90.6% of cases at doses ranging from 1.25 to 15 mg/day. The 27 patients who did not reach normal PRL values despite bromocriptine treatment at doses ranging from 15 to 60 mg administered orally for 3 months or more were characterized as bromocriptine-resistant. These 18 women and 9 men, aged 29 ± 9 years (mean ± SD, range 13–50) at the time of diagnosis had been followed up for 8 ± 4 years (2–16 years). The clinical and biological data from each patient were retrospectively reviewed. Hormone assays were performed using different commercial radioimmunoassay kits. All PRL levels represent the mean of at least 2 consecutive measurements. Normal PRL values were <25 μg/l in women and <17 μg/l in men. Each patient initially underwent evaluation of pituitary function by static and dynamic testing. The latter included measurements of plasma PRL in response to TRH (200 μg i.v.) and metoclopramide 2.5 mg i.v.), and of plasma LH and FSH response to GnRH (100 μg i.v.). These studies allowed to exclude hypersecretion of other pituitary hormones and to assess pituitary functions.

Results

Baseline Endocrine Status (table 1)

Presenting endocrine symptoms in the 18 women were amenorrhea-galactorrhea (n = 11), isolated secondary (n = 4) or primary (n = 2) amenorrhea, galactorrhea and secondary infertility (n = 1). All 9 men suffered from hypogonadism and 3 of them had hypopituitarism. Endocrine symptoms were already present 3.8 ± 3 years before diagnosis. Neuroradiological examinations (tomodensitometry and/or magnetic resonance imaging) revealed a microadenoma in 6 women and in none of the men. All but 1 man had macroadenomas with supra- or laterosellar extension, as did 44% of the women. Mean baseline PRL levels were 2,295 ± 562 μg/l (± SE) in the whole population. In keeping with tumor size, basal PRL concentrations were significantly higher in men (4,772 ± 1,126 μg/l) than in women (1,056 ± 394 μg/l).

Therapeutic Sequence (table 1)

Bromocriptine was the first treatment in 67% of these patients, including the 6 women harboring a microadenoma. Dopamine agonists represented the only treatment administered throughout the follow-up period in 5 of the microadenomas and in 1 macroadenoma. In the remaining patients, dopamine agonist treatment had to be combined to surgical or radiation therapies. In 8 cases, repetitive surgical treatments were necessary (up to 3 operations in 3 patients) due to further tumor growth after partial surgical removal of the tumor. Transfrontal route was used in 7 patients and had to be repeated in 1 of the cases. As a whole, 9 patients necessitated the 3 different therapeutic approaches.

Effects of the Dopamine Agonist Therapies (table 2)

During bromocriptine treatment all women remained amenorrheic and PRL levels were not decreased into the normal range despite gradual increase in drug doses up to 15–60 mg daily. Mean maximal suppression of PRL was 61 ± 8% (± SE) on bromocriptine and mean nadir PRL concentration on maximal doses of the drug were 240 ± 90 μg/l. A moderate decrease in tumor size (by ≤20%) was obtained in 3 patients while a further tumor growth was observed in 37% of these patients on bromocriptine therapy which motivated a complementary surgical and/or radiation therapy.

In the 9 patients who were shifted from oral to long-acting injectable bromocriptine, this formulation of the drug did not allow to normalize PRL levels. Fourteen days after a single 50-mg injection of long-acting repeatable bromocriptine, PRL levels had been reduced by <50% in 6 of these 9 resistant subject, as did only 2 of 33 (6%) macroprolactinoma patients normally responsive to bromocriptine treatment (their elevated PRL concentrations were suppressed to normal on long-term bromocriptine therapy). A poor inhibitory response 14 days after bromocriptine LAR injection could thus be considered as predictive of this resistance phenomenon. Nevertheless a marked initial PRL suppression (decrease in PRL levels by 68–76%) was also observed in patients who subsequently appeared as bromocriptine-resistant. No other initial feature could be identified as a possible predictor of bromocriptine resistance.

Table 1. Endocrine status, tumor mass and successive treatments in 27 prolactinoma patients resistant to bromocriptine

Patient No.	Sex	Age	Endocrine symptoms	Initial tumor mass	Basal PRL levels, μg/l[1]		Therapeutic sequence[2]	Follow-up years
					initial	after surgery		
1	F	34	A, G	micro	49	no surgery	BC, CV	13
2	F	19	A, G	micro	50	no surgery	BC, CV	12
3	F	26	A, G	micro	90	no surgery	BC, CV	4
4	F	27	A, G	micro	100	no surgery	BC, CV	8
5	F	23	A, G	macro	145	35	BC, TS, BC, R, CV	8
6	F	24	A, G	macro+SSE	146	96	BC, TS, BC, CV	4
7	F	29	A, G	micro	189	no surgery	BC, CV	8
8	F	15	A, G	micro	235	42	BC, TS, BC, TS, BC, CV	8
9	F	27	A, G	macro	250	180	BC, TS, BC, CV, BC	16
10	F	26	A, G	macro	328	211	BC, TS, BC, CV	5
11	M	33	hypogonadism	macro	350	51	TS, BC, CV	14
12	F	37	A	macro + LSE	350	220	BC, TS, BC, CV	7
13	F	21	A	macro + SSE + LSE	480	100	BC, TS, TF, R, BC, R, CV	8
14	F	31	A	macro	542	50	BC, TS, BC	15
15	M	34	hypogonadism	macro + SSE	600	125	TS, BC, TS, CV, TF, R, CV	9
16	F	17	primary A	macro + SSE	1,300	1000	TS, BC, R, BC	9
17	M	43	hypogonadism	macro + SSE	1,700	no surgery	BC, CV	2
18	F	46	A, G	macro + SSE	1,800	1,100	TS, R, BC, TF, BC, R, BC, TF, BC	8
19	F	25	A	macro + SSE	2,385	650	BC, CV, TS, CV	4
20	M	32	hypogonadism	macro + SSE	3,360	1,062	TS, BC, CV	6
21	F	13	hypopituitarism, G	macro + SSE	5,100	1,400	TF, BC, TS, BC, TS, BC, R, BC	7
22	F	23	primary A	macro + SSE	5,468	4,200	BC, TF, TS, BC, R, CV	5
23	M	50	hypogonadism	macro + SSE	5,500	1,526	TS, BC, CV	3
24	M	37	hypopituitarism	macro + SSE	6,500	no surgery	BC, R, CV	10
25	M	35	hypopituitarism	macro + SSE + LSE	7,500	2,500	BC, CV, TS, TF, R, CV	3
26	M	15	hypopituitarism	macro + SSE + LSE	8,110	1,450	TS, BC, CV	5
27	M	35	hypogonadism	macro + SSE + LSE	9,330	1,620	TS, TF, BC, CV, R, CV	14

F = Female; M = male; age = age at time of diagnosis; A = amenorrhea; G = galactorrhea; micro = microadenoma; macro = macroadenoma; SSE = suprasellar extension; LSE = laterosellar extension.

[1] Basal PRL levels (μg/l) are provided before any treatment (initial) and after the last surgical approach performed (after surgery).

[2] The different therapies used in each patient, listed in chronological order, include: transfrontal (TF) or transphenoidal (TS) surgery, oral and/or parenteral bromocriptine treatment (BC), CV 205-502 (CV) and pituitary roentgen therapy (R).

When we examined the long-term follow-up of these bromocriptine-resistant patients, we tried to determine whether such a resistance phenomenon appeared primarily or secondarily. Among the 14 patients who had been treated for 4 consecutive years or more by bromocriptine, a very partial suppression of PRL hypersecretion was observed in 8 of them (fig. 1a) from the beginning of the treatment, whereas the remaining patients were characterized by a secondary resistance phenomenon as illustrated in figure 1b.

Following unsuccessful bromocriptine treatment, 24 of the 27 patients were treated with the nonergot dopamine agonist CV 205-502. Half of them (9 women, 3 men) resumed normal plasma PRL levels and gonadal function on doses ranging from 150 to 450 μg daily. Despite relatively high daily doses of CV 205-502 (300–525 μg), the other patients were not normalized by this drug and 4 of them experienced ongoing tumor growth while on therapy, as detailed in table 2. On the contrary, in 4 other patients this drug was able to induce a clear-cut tumor shrinkage (by 40% or more). During CV 205-502 treatment, mean maximal inhibition of PRL hypersecretion was 66 ± 7% (± SE) and mean nadir PRL concentration achieved was 72 ± 31 μg/l.

Table 2. Effects of the dopamine agonist therapies bromocriptine and CV 205-502 in 24 of the 27 bromocriptine-resistant patients treated with both drugs successively

Patient No.	On bromocriptine			On CV 205–502		
	dose[1] mg/day	PRL[2] µg/l	change in tumor size[3]	dose[1] µg/day	PRL[2] µg/l	change in tumor size[3]
1	15	40	0	150	4	0
2	15	27	0	300	45	0
3	15	25	0	450	18	0
4	30	28	0	300	19	0
5	15	43	growth	300	6	0
6	15	38	–20%	300	18	0
7	15	60	0	300	18	0
8	15	36	growth	500	30	0
9	15	25	0	300	35	0
10	15	45	0	300	35	0
11	15	32	0	300	12	0
12	15	170	0	300	90	0
13	60	42	growth	300	10	growth
14	30	25	0	300	25	0
15	15	59	growth	500	90	growth
17	15	100	–20%	300	37	–40%
19	15	110	–10%	300	15	–40%
20	30	675	0	500	510	0
22	30	80	growth	300	24	0
23	15	226	0	525	25	–7%
24	30	32	growth	150	18	–42%
25	15	2,200	growth	500	600	growth
26	15	250	0	300	20	–72%
27	30	97	growth	400	30	growth

[1] Maximal daily doses for bromocriptine (given t.i.d.) and CV 205-502 (administered once daily at bedtime) are given in mg and µg, respectively.
[2] Nadir PRL concentratons (µg/l) represent the lowest PRL level achieved while on maximal daily dose of each drug.
[3] Percentage change in tumor size represents the maximal decrease in the largest diameter of the tumor as measured on similar sections of consecutive pituitary computerized tomography scans.

Overall Outcome

In terms of overall outcome, 2 female patients (No. 13 and 18) deceased from invasive cerebral extensions of their tumor, the former having a MEN type 1. In a third patient (No. 15) with a very invasive tumor, the observation of vertebral metastases with positive anti-PRL immunostaining led to the diagnosis of malignant prolactinoma. Among the women who resumed normal (n = 9) or near normal PRL levels (n = 4) on CV 205-502 treatment, 6 obtained a spontaneous pregnancy. Finally, 2 women with posttherapeutic hypopituitarism could be considered as cured of their resistant prolactinoma 5 and 6 years after surgery and radiotherapy.

Discussion

Our group and others have underlined the variety of responses to dopamine and its agonists which have been observed both in vivo and in cultured prolactinoma cells [3, 14, 16]. The data from the literature suggest that several sites in the dopamine – D_2 receptor – second messenger pathways may be involved in such a resistance phenomenon. Indeed, in a previous study we had evidenced a decrease in D_2 dopamine receptor sites in some of the adenomatous lactotrophs from bromocriptine-resistant prolactinoma patients [14]. The fact that a more potent D_2 dopamine agonist such as CV 205-502 was able to overcome this resistance phenomenon in only a fraction

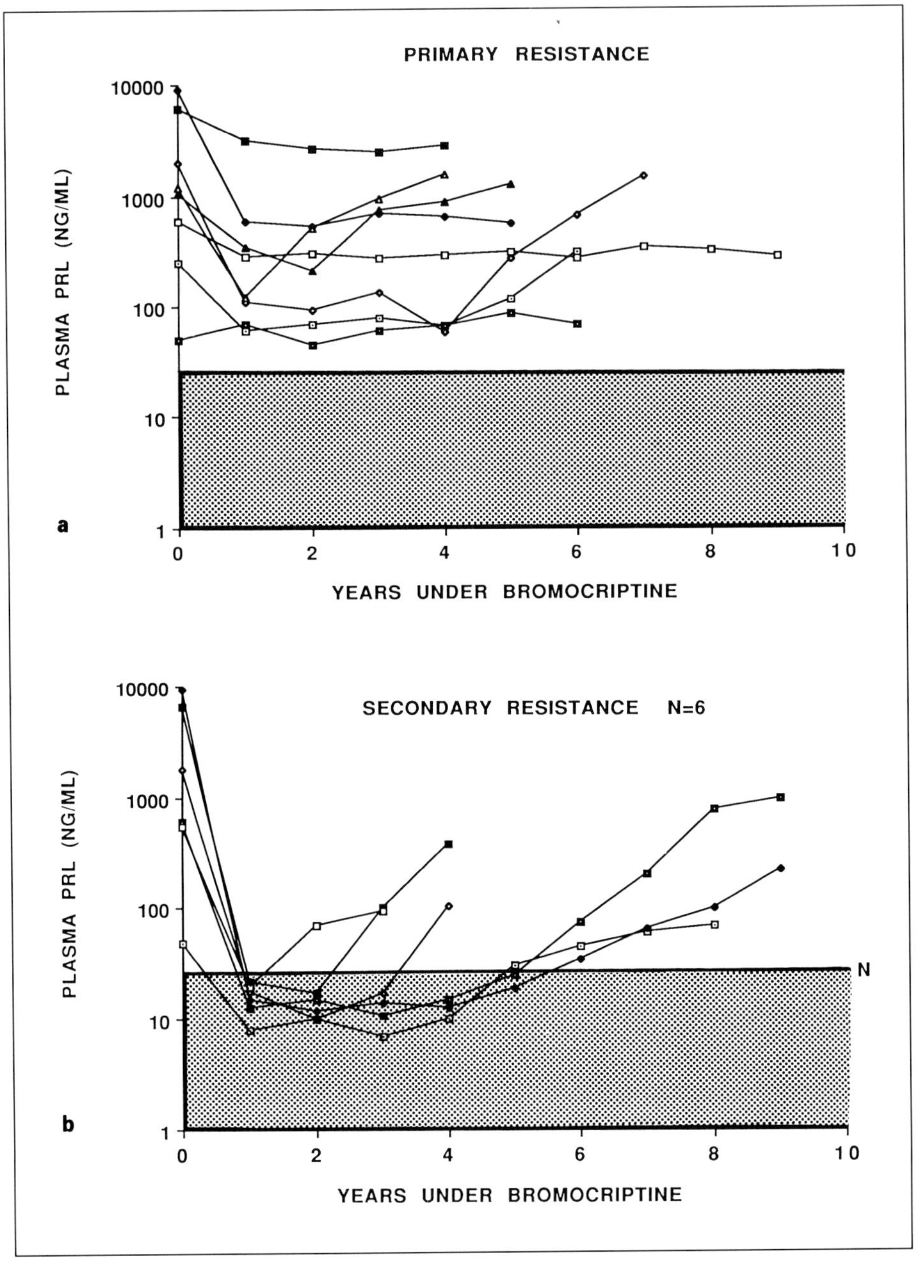

Fig. 1. Time course of PRL levels in 14 bromocriptine-resistant patients treated by this drug for at least 4 consecutive years. In 8 of them, each represented in figure 1a by a different symbol, a primary resistance was diagnosed as their plasma PRL levels remained above the upper limit of normal range (shaded area) throughout the whole treatment period. In contrast, in the 6 remaining patients, represented in figure 1b by a distinct symbol, PRL levels were normalized during the first year of treatment and increased above normal range (N, shaded area) despite dose adjustment, 1–6 years after the start of the treatment.

of such patients [16, 17] suggests that postreceptor defects might also be involved. A highly invasive prolactinoma has recently been shown to be associated with a mutation in codon 12 of the H-ras gene [18]. In the future, similar approaches will probably shed more light on the pathophysiology of pituitary neoplasia. Further studies are warranted to determine the abnormalities involved in each individual case.

Whatever the mechanism underlying the resistance to dopamine agonists, it was the aim of the present study to describe more precisely the clinical outcome of these patients. Although prolactinomas, even those with large and aggressive tumors, can nowadays be dealt with in the majority of cases with minimal morbidity [19, 20], the bromocriptine-resistant prolactinomas represent the most severe aspect of this disease. They necessitate in most cases a combination of medical, neurosurgical and radiation therapies which are not always able to prevent a fatal outcome.

References

1 Besser GM, Parke L, Edwards CR, et al: Galactorrhea: Successful treatment with reduction of plasma prolactin levels by bromoergocryptine. BMJ 1972;iii:669–672.
2 MacLeod RM, Lehmeyer JE: Studies on the mechanism of the dopamine mediated inhibition of prolactin secretion. Endocrinology 1974;94:1077–1085.
3 Wood DF, Johnston JM, Johnston DG: Dopamine, the dopamine D_2 receptor and pituitary tumours (Review). Clin Endocrinol 1991;35: 455–466.
4 Molitch ME, Elton RL, Blackwell RO, et al. Bromocriptine as primay therapy for prolactin-secreting macroadenomas: Results of a prospective multicenter study. J Clin Endocrinol Metab 1985;60:698–705.
5 Grossman A, Bouloux PMG, Loneragan R, et al: Comparison of the clinical activity of mesulergine and pergolide in the treatment of hyperprolactinemia. Clin Endocrinol 1986;22: 611–616.
6 Ferrari C, Barbieri C, Caldara R, et al: Long-lasting prolactin-lowering effect of cabergoline, a new dopamine agonist, in hyperprolactinemic patients. J Clin Endocrinol Metab 1986; 63:941–945.
7 Khalfallah Y, Claustrat B, Grochowicki M, et al: Effects of a new prolactin inhibitor, CV 205-502, in the treatment of human macroprolactinomas. J Clin Endocrinol Metab 1990;71:354–359.
8 Brue T, Lancranjan I, Louvet JP, et al: A long-acting repeatable form of bromocriptine as long-term treatment of prolactin-secreting macroadenomas: A multicenter study. Fertil Steril 1992;57:74–80.
9 Thorner MO, Schran HF, Evans WS, et al: A broad spectrum of prolactin suppression by bromocriptine in hyperprolactinemic women: A study of serum prolactin and bromocriptine levels after acute and chronic administration of bromocriptine. J Clin Endocrinol Metab 1980; 50:1026–1033.
10 Borenstein R, Kessler I, Ben David M: Prolactin resistance to bromocryptine treatment. A case report. Int J Fertil 1981;26:287–289.
11 Wass JAH, Williams J, Charleworth M, et al: Bromocriptine in management of large pituitary tumors. BMJ 1982;284:1908–1911.
12 Johnston DG, Prescott RWG, Kendall-Taylor P, et al: Hyperprolactinemia. Long-term effects of bromocriptine. Am J Med 1983;75:868–874.
13 Kuhn JM, Gancel A, Weinstein A, et al: Traitement médical des adénomes hypophysaires à prolactine. Presse Méd 1985;14:525–528.
14 Pellegrini I, Rasolonjanahary R, Gunz G, et al: Resistance to bromocriptine in prolactinomas. J Clin Endocrinol Metab 1989;69:500–509.
15 Davis JRE, Sheppard MC, Heath DA: Giant invasive prolactinoma: A case report and review of nine further cases. Q J Med 1990;74: 227–238.
16 Brue T, Pellegrini I, Gunz G, et al. Effects of the dopamine agonist CV 205-502 in human prolactinomas resistant to bromocriptine. J Clin Endocrinol Metab 1992;74:577–584.
17 Duranteau L, Chanson P, Lavoinne A, et al: Effect of the new dopaminergic agonist CV 205-502 on plasma prolactin levels and tumour size in bromocriptine-resistant prolactinomas. Clin Endocrinol 1991;34:25–29.
18 Karga HJ, Alexander JM, Hedley-White ET, et al: Ras mutations in human pituitary tumors. J Clin Endocrinol Metab 1992;74:914–919.
19 Grossman A: The modern management of macroprolactinomas. Trends Endocrinol Metab 1991;2:163–168.
20 Bevan JS, Webster J, Burke CW, Scanlon MF: Dopamine agonists and pituitary tumor shrinkage. Endocr Rev 1992;13:220–240.

Horm Res 1992;38:90–93

Anna Spada[a]
Lucia Vallar[b]

[a] Institute of Endocrine Sciences, Ospedale Maggiore IRCCS and
[b] Department of Pharmacology, CNR Center of Cytopharmacology, Scientific Institute San Raffaele, University of Milan, Italy

G-Protein Oncogenes in Acromegaly

Abstract

G-proteins belong to a family of proteins which share the common properties of GTP binding and hydrolysis. Heterotrimeric G-proteins are composed of α-, β- and γ-subunits. The α-subunit which differs from one G-protein to another contains the GDP/GTP binding site and has intrinsic GTPase activity. The receptor occupancy causes displacement of bound GDP by GTP, dissociation of free βγ-dimer and α-GTP complex, interaction of the activated α-GTP complex with intracellular effectors, such as enzymes and ion channels. The turn off of the reaction is due to the GTPase activity which causes the hydrolysis of GTP to GDP. G-proteins are essential for transferring hormonal signals from cell surface receptors to intracellular effectors. Since G-proteins generate intracellular effectors involved in cell growth, G-protein genes have the propensity to be converted into oncogenes. In fact, mutations in the α-subunit of Gs (the G-protein involved in the activation of adenylyl cyclase) have been demonstrated in 40% of human GH secreting pituitary adenomas. Single amino acid substitutions replacing Arg 201 with either Cys or His or Gln 227 with either Arg or Leu cause constitutive activation of adenylyl cyclase by inhibiting GTPase (*gsp* oncogene). The same mutations were identified in about 10% of thyroid adenomas and in the McCune-Albright syndrome.

Key Words
G-proteins
Oncogene
Adenylyl cyclase
cAMP
Acromegaly
GH-secreting pituitary adenomas

Introduction

Heterotrimeric G-proteins belong to a large family of proteins which share the common properties of GTP binding and hydrolysis. G-proteins are essential for transferring hormonal signals from cell surface receptors to intracellular effectors. In fact, a variety of hormones, neurotransmitters and growth factors requires the presence of receptors able to recognize and activate G-proteins which subsequently generate intracellular effector molecules. Up to the present time, 30 or more G-protein-coupled receptors have been cloned and it is easily predictable that this number will increase in the near future [1–6]. By molecular cloning, G-protein-coupled receptors have been demonstrated to belong to a large family of proteins characterized by seven hydrophobic α-helices [7–10]. Site-directed mutagenesis and deletion analysis have been utilized to determine structure/function relationships. An increasing body of evidence points to the transmembrane domains as important in forming the ligand-binding site while the third cytoplasmatic loop and to a limited extent the carboxyl-terminal end have been proposed to contain major recognition sites for G-proteins [11, 12].

G-Proteins

Heterotrimeric G-proteins are composed of α-, β- and γ-subunits [13–18]. The functional specificity of each G-protein is due to the α-subunit, which differs from one G-protein to another while β- and γ-subunits are functionally interchangeable among different G-proteins. The α-subunit also contains the GDP/GTP binding site and has intrinsic GTPase activity. The receptor occupancy causes

Anna Spada, MD
Institute of Endocrine Sciences, Pad. Granelli
Ospedale Maggiore IRCCS
via F. Sforza 35
I-20122 Milano (Italy)

conformational changes of the α-subunit leading to displacement of bound GDP by GTP. After GTP binding, G-proteins undergo a dissociation reaction resulting in free βγ-dimers and α-GTP complexes. The α-subunit GTP complex is the activated form of G-protein since this molecule is effective in regulating the activity of intracellular effectors, such as specific enzymes and ion channels. In addition, the α-subunit possesses an intrinsic GTPase activity which causes the hydrolysis of α-GTP to α-GDP, thus ensuring the turn-off of the reaction.

Through purification and molecular cloning techniques, more than 20 distinct vertebrate α-subunits and multiple β- and γ-subunits have been identified.

G-Protein Oncogenes

Many proto-oncogenes encode proteins that transmit signals regulating normal cell functions. Specific mutations convert these genes into oncogenes, whose products are responsible for the abnormal growth of malignant cells. Since G-proteins generate intracellular effectors which are also involved in cell growth, G-protein genes have the propensity to be converted into oncogenes. Accordingly, oncogenic mutations of G-proteins have been recently identified in human endocrine disorders (table 1) [19–24].

Table 1. G-protein oncogenes in human diseases

G-protein	Oncogene	Disease	Reference
Gs	*gsp*	Acromegaly	20, 21
		McCune-Albright	24
		Thyroid adenomas	23
		Thyroid tumors	22
Gi2	*gip2*	Ovary tumors	21
		Adrenal tumors	21

Gsp Oncogene in Acromegaly

Activating Mutations in Human GH-Secreting Adenomas

GH secretion is dually regulated by GH-releasing hormone (GHRH) and somatostatin (SRIH) which exert a stimulatory and inhibitory action, respectively. GHRH interacts with a specific receptor coupled to Gs, leading to the stimulation of adenylyl cyclase (AC) and cAMP accumulation. SRIH activates a more complex pattern of G-proteins, resulting in the inhibition of AC as well as reduction in cytosolic calcium concentrations, possibly due to K+ channels activation and membrane hyperpolarization [25–27].

Several lines of evidence indicate that the two hypothalamic peptides are involved in the control of both hormone release and cell replication, the two effects largely depending on cAMP modulation. In fact, it has been demonstrated that in normal somatotrophs cAMP exerts a proliferative action, although in several cell types cAMP induces differentiation. In in vitro experiments, GHRH was demonstrated to promote somatotroph proliferation by a cAMP-dependent mechanism, whereas evidence indicates that SRIH exerts an antiproliferative effect [28–30]. Moreover, the recent observation that the targeted expression by cholera toxin produces somatotroph hyperplasia and gigantism in transgenic mice further support the hypothesis that somatotrophs are cells programmed to proliferate in response to elevated cAMP levels [31].

As a general rule, tumoral somatotrophs express receptors for both GHRH and SRIH which display a normal coupling with the appropriate G-protein. However, in recent years a subset of GH-secreting adenomas characterized by high levels of in vitro GH release, membrane AC activity and intracellular cAMP accumulation even under unstimulated conditions was identified [19]. The constitutive activation of AC in these tumors was proved to be due to the presence of mutations in the α-subunit of Gs. Single amino acid substitutions replaced Arg 201 with either Cys of His or Gln 227 with either Arg or Leu [20, 21]. Genomic DNA from peripheral blood cells contained only wild-type sequence, in keeping with the view of a somatic origin of αs mutations. Mutations at both Arg 201 and Gln 227 were proved to produce proteins with very low GTPase activity in the transfected cells [20]. Indeed, both amino acid residues replaced by these mutations were already known or suspected to be important in GTP hydrolysis since Arg 201 is the residue ADP-ribosylated by cholera toxin, a covalent modification inhibiting GTPase, while Gln 227 is located in the presumed guanine nucleotide binding region of αs, at a position corresponding to Gln 61 of p21 *ras*. Therefore, the mutations stabilize αs in its active conformation, thus mimicking the effect of specific extracellular growth factors, such as GHRH. The screening of a large number of GH-secreting adenomas showed that mutations occur in about 40% of the tumors tested [21].

The identification of mutations that activate αs by inhibiting GTPase in human pituitary tumors led to the

Table 2. Characteristics of GH-secreting tumors with *gsp* oncogene

In vitro
High GH release (ng/30 min/2^5 cells: 53 ± 12 in group 1[1] versus 250 ± 78 in group 2[2])
High cAMP levels (pmol/2^5 cells: 2.2 ± 0.1 in group 1 versus 50 ± 16 in group 2)
High AC-activity (pmol cAMP/mg/min: 12 ± 2 in group 1 versus 130 ± 22 in group 2)
At electron microscopy, densely granulated cells
In vivo
High plasma GH levels (μg/l: 32 ± 33 in group 1 versus 45 ± 35 in group 2)
Poor sensitivity to GHRH (% net increase: 186 ± 220 in group 1 versus 79 ± 80 in group 2)
High sensitivity to SRIH (% net decrease: 63 ± 18 in group 1 versus 79 ± 9 in group 2)
High frequency of microadenomas

Materials and Methods were as described in Vallar et al. [19] and Spada et al. [33].
1 Group 1: tumors without *gsp* oncogene.
2 Group 2: tumors with *gsp* oncogene.

proposal that the αs gene can be converted into an oncogene, designate *gsp* (for Gs protein) in cells programmed to proliferate in response to cAMP.

Clinical, Biochemical and Morphological Correlates in Patients with gsp *Oncogene*

Clinical and biochemical parameters were evaluated in patients with pituitary tumors expressing *gsp* mutations. No difference in age, sex, clinical features, duration of the disease or cure rate was observed between patients with and without *gsp* oncogene [32, 33]. Patients with *gsp* oncogene were reported to have tumors small in size which sustained high circulating GH levels [33]. The hypersecretory state was confirmed by the morphological features of these tumors, which were characterized by the presence of densely granulated cells with well-developed RER and prominent Golgi complex. In agreement with the in vitro data, patients with *gsp* oncogene were poorly sensitive to GHRH administration while they were extremely sensitive to the inhibitory action of both SRIH and dopamine (table 2). These data suggest that the expression of oncogenic mutations might be at least partially counteracted by inhibitory agents and this might account for the low progression of the disease, independently of the presence of *gsp* oncogene.

Gsp *Oncogene in the McCune-Albright Syndrome*

Acromegaly is frequently present in patients affected with the McCune-Albright syndrome [34, 35]. This syndrome is a rare disease characterized by polyostotic fibrous dysplasia, pigmentation of the skin and multiple endocrinopathies which include, in addition to acromegaly, sexual precocity, hyperthyroidism and adrenal hyperfunction. The observation that these endocrine tissues are sensitive to trophic agents which activate cAMP production have led to the hypothesis that a constitutive activation of this enzyme may play a role in the pathogenesis of the disease. In a very recent study, *gsp* oncogene was found in several tissues from 4 patients with McCune-Albright syndrome [24]. Activating mutations, replacing Arg 201 with either His or Cys, were found in the affected organs as well as in tissues not classically involved in the disease. Since *gsp* oncogene was absent in at least one tissue from each patient, indicating the somatic origin of the mutations, the authors conclude that the McCune-Albright syndrome is due to an early postzygotic *gsp* mutation resulting in mosaicism [24]. The presence of this oncogene and the constitutive activation of cAMP formation may account for the hyperplasia of several tissues constituted by cells programmed to proliferate in response to cAMP.

Conclusions

It has long been known that proteins involved in the signalling system are possible targets for oncogenic mutations. In fact, several oncogene products mimic the effects of ligands, receptors and regulatory enzymes. Naturally occurring mutations of GTP-binding proteins have been up to very recently identified exclusively in p21 *ras* genes. The recent identification of mutations in the α-subunit of heterotrimeric G-proteins dramatically expand the potential role of these proteins. Although *gsp* oncogene has been identified in rare diseases such as acromegaly and the McCune-Albright syndrome, it has been proposed that *gsp* oncogene might be present in other tissues in which cAMP exerts a proliferative effect. This hypothesis has been confirmed by the recent observation that *gsp* mutations are present in a good proportion of thyroid autonomous functioning adenomas and differentiated thyroid tumors [22, 23]. This finding is in agreement with the well-known proliferative role exerted by cAMP in thyroid cells [36, 37].

As far as the presence of mutations in other G-proteins is concerned, mutations of the α-subunit of Gi2 have been recently identified in tumors of the ovary and adrenal cortex (*gip2* oncogene [21]). Since the intracellular effectors triggered by Gi2 are multiple (inhibition of AC, activation of K+ channels, reduction of cytosolic calcium) and probably not completely understood, the oncogenic potential of constitutive activation of Gi2 is yet to be identified.

Finally, it is easily predictable that mutations converting other G-protein genes into oncogenes will be identified in the near future.

References

1 Dixon RAF, Kobilka BK, Strader DJ, Benovig SL, Dohlmana HG, Frielle T, Polanowski MA, Bennett CD, Rands E, Dienl RE, Mumford RA, Slater EE, Sigal IS, Caron MC, Lefkowitz R, Strader CD: Cloning of the gene and cDNA for mammalian β-adrenergic receptor and homology with rhodopsin. Nature 1986;321:75–79.

2 Nathans J, Hodness DS: Isolation, sequence analysis and intron-exon arrangement of the gene encoding bovine rhodopsin. Cell 1983;34:807–811.

3 Kobilka BK, Matsui H, Kobilka TS, Yang-Feng TL, Francke V, Caron MG, Lefkowitz RJ, Regan JW: Cloning, sequencing and expression of the gene coding for the human platelet α_2-adrenergic receptor. Science 1987;238:650–656.

4 Kubo T, Fakuda K, Mikami A, Maeda A, Takabashi H, Miolina M, Haga T, Haga K, Idiyama A, Kangawa K, Kojima M, Matsao H, Hirose T, Numa S: Cloning, sequencing and expression of complementary DNA encoding the muscarinic acetylcholine receptor. Nature 1986;323:411–416.

5 Masu Y, Nakayama K, Tamaki H, Harada Y, Kuno M, Nakanishi S: cDNA cloning of bovine substance-K receptor through oocyte expression system. Nature 1987;329:836–838.

6 Parmentier M, Libert F, Maenhaut C, Lefort A, Gerard C, Perret J, Van Sande S, Dumont JE, Vassart G: Molecular cloning of the thyrotropin receptor. Science 1989;246:1620–1622.

7 Dohlman HG, Caron MG, Lefkowitz RJ: A family of receptors coupled to guanine nucleotide regulatory proteins. Biochemistry 1987;26:2657–2663.

8 Lefkowitz RJ, Caron MG: Adrenergic receptors; models for the study of receptors coupled to guanine nucleotide regulatory proteins. J Biol Chem 1988;263:4993–4996.

9 Findlay J, Eliopoulos E: Three-dimensional modelling of G-protein linked receptors. Trends Pharmacol Sci 1990;11:492–499.

10 Strosberg AD: Structure/function relationship of proteins belonging to the family of receptors coupled to GTP binding proteins. Eur Biochem 1991;196:1–10.

11 Frielle T, Daniel K, Caron MG, Lefkowitz RJ: Structural basis of β-adrenoceptor subtype specifically based upon chimeric β_1-β_2-adrenoceptors. Proc Natl Acad Sci USA 1988;85:9494–9498.

12 Kobilka BK, Kobilka TS, Daniel K, Regan JW, Caron MG, Lefkowitz RJ: Chimeric α_2-β_2-adrenergic receptors: Delineation of domains involved in effector coupling and ligand binding specificity. Science 1988;240:1310–1316.

13 Sryer L, Bourne H: G-proteins: A family of signal transducers. Annu Rev Cell Biol 1986;2:391–419.

14 Gilman AG: G-proteins: Transducers of receptor-generated signals. Annu Rev Biochem 1987;56:615–649.

15 Johnson GL, Dhanasekaran N: The G-protein family and their interaction with receptors. Endocrine Rev 1989;10:317–331.

16 Bourne HR, Sanders DA, McCormick F: The GTPase superfamily: A conserved switch for diverse cell functions. Nature 1990;348:125–132.

17 Birnbaumer L, Abramowitz J, Brown AM: Receptor-effector coupling by G-proteins. Biochim Biophys Acta 1990;1031:163–224.

18 Simon MI, Strathmann MP, Gautam N: Diversity of G proteins in signal transduction. Science 1991;252:802–808.

19 Vallar L, Spada A, Giannattasio G: Altered Gs and adenylate cyclase activity in human GH-secreting pituitary adenomas. Nature 1987;330:566–568.

20 Landis CA, Masters SB, Spada A, Pace AM, Bourne HR, Vallar L: GTPase inhibiting mutations activate the α chain of Gs and stimulate adenylyl cyclase in human pituitary tumors. Nature 1989;340:692–696.

21 Lyons J, Landis CA, Harsh G, Vallar L, Grunewald K, Feichtinger H, Duh QY, Clark OH, Kawasaki E, Bourne HR, McCormick F: Two G-protein oncogenes in human endocrine tumors. Science 1990;249:655–659.

22 Suarez HG, Duvillard JA, Caillu B, Schlumberger M, Parmentier C, Monier R: *Gsp* mutations in human thyroid tumours. Oncogene 1991;6:677–679.

23 Osullivan C, Barton CM, Staddon SL, Brown CL, Lemoine NR: Activating point mutations in the *gsp* oncogene in human thyroid adenomas. Mol Carcinog 1991;4:345–349.

24 Weinstein LS, Shenker A, Gejman P, Marino MJ, Friedman E, Spiegel AM: Activating mutations of the stimulatory G protein in the McCune-Albright syndrome. N Engl J Med 1991;325:1688–1695.

25 Bilezikjian LM, Vale W: Stimulation of adenosine 3′,5′-monophosphate production by growth hormone-releasing factor and its inhibition by somatostatin in anterior pituitary cells in vitro. Endocrinology 1983;113;1726–1731.

26 Spada A, Vallar L, Giannattasio G: Presence of an adenylate cyclase dually regulated by somatostatina and human pancreatic growth hormone (GH)-releasing factor in GH-secreting cells. Endocrinology 1984;115:1203–1209.

27 Dorflinger L, Schonbrunn A: Somatostatin inhibits basal and vasoactive peptide stimulated release by different mechanisms in GH pituitary cells. Endocrinology 1983;113:1551–1558.

28 Billestrup N, Swanson LW, Vale W: Growth hormone releasing factor stimulates cell proliferation of somatotrophs in vitro. Proc Natl Acad Sci USA 1986;83:6854–6857.

29 Billestrup L, Mitchell RL, Vale W, Verma IM: Growth hormone releasing factor induces c-*fos* expression in cultured primary pituitary cells. Mol Endocrinol 1987;1:300–305.

30 Schally AV: Oncological applications of somatostatin analogues. Cancer Res 1988;48:6977–6985.

31 Burton FH, Hasel KW, Bloom FE, Sutcliffe JG: Pituitary hyperplasia and gigantism in mice caused by a cholera toxin transgene. Nature 1991;350:74–77.

32 Landis CA, Harsh G, Lyons J, Davis RL, McCormick F, Bourne HR: Clinic characteristics of acromegalic patients whose pituitary tumors contain mutant Gs protein. J Clin Endocrinol Metab 1990;71:1416–1420.

33 Spada A, Arosio M, Bochicchio D, Bazzoni N, Vallar L, Bassetti M, Faglia G: Clinical biochemical and morphological correlates in patients bearing growth hormone secreting tumors with or without constitutively active adenylyl cyclase. J Clin Endocrinol Metab 1990;71:1421–1426.

34 McCune DJ: Osteitis fibrosa cystica: The case of a nine-year-old girl who also exhibits precocious puberty, multiple pigmentation of the skin and hyperthyroidism. Am J Dis Child 1936;52:743–744.

35 Benedict PH: Endocrine features of Albright's syndrome. Acta Endocrinol (Copenh) 1986;11:30–45.

36 Dumont JE, Jauniaux JC, Roger PP: The cyclic AMP-mediated stimulation of cell proliferation. Trends Biochem Sci 1989;14:67–71.

37 Maenhaut C, Roger PP, Reuse S, Dumont JE: Activation of the cyclic AMP cascade as an oncogenic mechanism: The thyroid example. Biochimie 1991;73:29–36.

Horm Res 1992;38:94–99

Jérôme Bertherat[a]
Philippe Chanson[b]
Didier Dewailly[c]
Alain Enjalbert[a]
Philippe Jaquet[d]
Claude Kordon[a]
Françoise Peillon[e]
José Timsit[f]
Jacques Epelbaum[a]

[a] INSERM U.159, Centre Paul-Broca de l'INSERM, Paris;
[b] Hôpital Lariboisière, Paris;
[c] CHRU de Lille, Lille;
[d] Hôpital Nord, Marseille;
[e] INSERM U. 223, CHU Pitié-la-Salpêtrière, Paris;
[f] INSERM U. 25 Hôpital Necker, Paris, France

Resistance to Somatostatin (SRIH) Analog Therapy in Acromegaly

Re-Evaluation of the Correlation between the SRIH Receptor Status of the Pituitary Tumor and the in vivo Inhibition of GH Secretion in Response to SRIH Analog

Key Words
Acromegaly
Somatostatin receptor
Somatostatin analog
Adenylate cyclase

Abstract
The development of a long-acting somatostatin (SRIH) analog (octreotide, Sandoz) has been a major breakthrough in the treatment of acromegaly. However, in 20–30% of the patients, growth hormone (GH) plasma levels remain elevated (> 10 μg/l) despite treatment with octreotide. This raised the concept of resistance to SRIH analog therapy in acromegaly. Indeed, in vivo response to SRIH analogs varies greatly among acromegalic patients. According to the reviews in the literature and our own autoradiographic data, no direct correlation can be established between the GH response to octreotide and the number or affinity of the SRIH receptors located on the tumor. In our series a greater density of SRIH receptors is present on tumors from patients very sensitive to the SRIH agonist. A subset of patients resistant to octreotide could result from a very low density of SRIH receptor although this type of GH-secreting tumor constitutes certainly a rare case. A subset of GH-secreting pituitary tumors can be characterized by a mutation on the α subunit of the guanine nucleotide-dependent protein coupled to the stimulation of adenylate cyclase (Gαs). This mutation results in a high basal adenylate cyclase activity and a low GHRH-stimulated activity. However, when the adenomas are separated according to their basal adenylate cyclase activity, SRIH is able to decrease cAMP levels in both types of tumor. In addition, in our series no direct correlation is observed between the SRIH inhibition of adenylate cyclase and the amount of SRIH-binding sites. Taken together, these findings suggest that in addition to a lack of SRIH-binding sites on some rare octreotide-resistant GH-secreting tumors, other mechanisms could be involved in the differential sensitivity to SRIH analogs.

Introduction

The tetradecapeptide somatostatin (SRIH) was discovered as an inhibitory neurohormone decreasing growth hormone (GH) secretion from anterior pituitary cells [1]. The most obvious clinical application of this finding was the treatment of acromegaly and less than 1 year after its discovery, it was reported that SRIH is able to decrease GH plasma levels in acromegalic patients [2, 3]. In vitro studies of GH-secreting pituitary adenomas demon-

J. Epelbaum
INSERM U. 159
2ter, rue d'Alésia
F-75014 Paris (France)

strated a direct inhibitory effect of SRIH on GH secretion [4, 5]. This effect is mediated through specific SRIH receptors characterized on rat somatotrophs [6] as well as on GH-secreting adenomas [7–9]. The action of SRIH on pituitary somatotrophs is mediated through multiple mechanisms involving the inhibition of adenylate cyclase [10–12], the opening of K^+ channels [13] and the subsequent closing of voltage-dependent Ca^{2+} channels [14].

Originally, the variability of in vivo, as well as in vitro, GH response to SRIH in GH-secreting pituitary tumors [2, 5, 15] was attributed to the very short half-life of the native peptide. The development of potent long-acting SRIH analogs was of major importance in the treatment of acromegaly [for review, see 16]. Nevertheless, patients with GH-secreting adenomas showed a heterogeneity in the response of plasma GH levels to SRIH analog administration [16]. Increasing the daily dose of SRIH analog [17], or the use of subcutaneous infusion [18], did not lead to normalization of GH plasma levels in all patients. It was thus postulated that the heterogeneity of GH inhibition could be related to differences in SRIH receptor densities [19, 20]. In addition, in a subset of GH-secreting pituitary tumors, a mutation of the α_s subunit of G protein that constitutively activates adenylate cyclase has been reported [21, 22]. It was therefore suggested that GH-secreting adenomas with high basal adenylate cyclase activity are more sensitive to SRIH [23].

In this review, in parallel with our own results concerning patients with GH-secreting adenomas, we shall summarize studies concerning the in vivo effect of SRIH agonists on GH plasma levels in acromegaly and the characterization of SRIH receptors, as well as the effect of SRIH on adenylate cyclase in pituitary and GH-secreting adenomas. Finally, we shall compare the in vivo sensitivity of GH to SRIH analogs and the receptor status of the adenomas.

Effects of the SRIH Agonist Octreotide on GH Plasma Levels in Acromegaly

There is a close correlation between the GH decrease during an acute injection of octreotide and the long-term response to this treatment [24]. However, the concept of SRIH agonist resistance in acromegaly derives from chronic studies.

In a review including 377 patients treated with octreotide [16], a decrease in GH plasma levels below 5 µg/l was observed in 55% of the patients, while GH plasma levels remained above 10 µg/l in 22% of the cases. Despite the different therapeutic regimens used by the various investigators, similar percentages of patients – very sensitive to octreotide on the one side and resistant on the other – were reported in most studies. More recently, in 58 acromegalic patients [17], it was shown that, with an incremental dose protocol, GH plasma levels are normalized in 22% of the patients, improved in 56% and unchanged in 22%. Even when using a continuous subcutaneous infusion of octreotide, the variability in GH response and resistance to SRIH agonist therapy are observed [18, 25]. In a European multicenter study, involving 178 patients, it was suggested that a 3 times daily administration of 100 µg octreotide was the mean optimal dose [26]. In order to define the mechanisms of the sensitivity to octreotide in acromegaly, we studied the GH plasma level response to a single subcutaneous injection of 100 µg in 15 patients before surgical removal of the GH-secreting tumor. Plasma GH levels decreased by more than 80% from basal levels in 33% of the patients, from 50 to 80% in 27% of the patients and by less than 50% in 40% of the patients which were considered as resistant to octreotide.

Characterization of SRIH Receptor on Pituitary Cells and GH-Secreting Pituitary Adenomas

Binding Studies

Since the original study of Schonbrunn and Tashjian [6] on a clonal pituitary cell line, numerous authors have described the properties of nanomolar affinity SRIH-binding sites in pituitary [27–30]. Various monoiodinated tyrosine-substituted SRIH agonists bind, in saturation experiments, to a single class of binding sites. ^{125}I-SRIH binding is positively regulated by divalent cations [28] and negatively by guanine nucleotides [31]. The latter findings strongly suggest that SRIH-binding sites are coupled to guanine-nucleotide- and magnesium-binding proteins which are involved in cAMP- and/or calcium-dependent transducing mechanisms.

In pituitary tumors high but variable densities of ^{125}I-SRIH-binding sites are measured in GH-secreting adenomas [7–9], and, to a lesser extent, in TSH-secreting adenomas [32, 33]. Similarly, among ten TSH-secreting adenomas, the highest ^{125}I-SRIH-binding site densities were found on the two mixed GH/TSH adenomas [32, 33]. ^{125}I-SRIH-binding sites are much less numerous or even undetectable in the case of prolactinomas (fig. 1) and in nonfunctioning pituitary tumors [7–9, 33]. In pure GH-secreting adenomas, ^{125}I-SRIH-binding site density, studied on membrane preparations, varies 10-fold in indi-

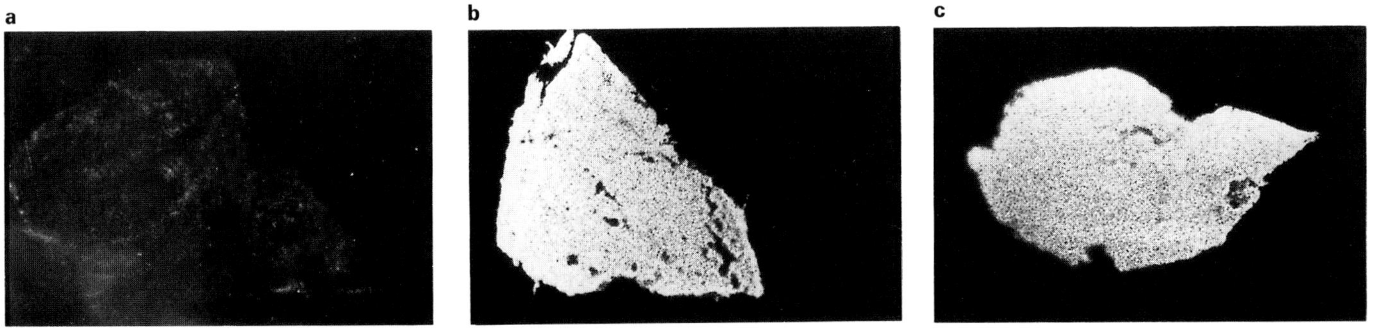

Fig. 1. Autoradiograms of ^{125}I-SRIH-binding sites in pituitary adenomas. Total binding in a PRL-secreting adenoma (**a**) with low binding site density, in a GH-secreting adenoma (**b**) with high density of ^{125}I-SRIH-binding sites and in a mixed GH/PRL pituitary tumor (**c**).

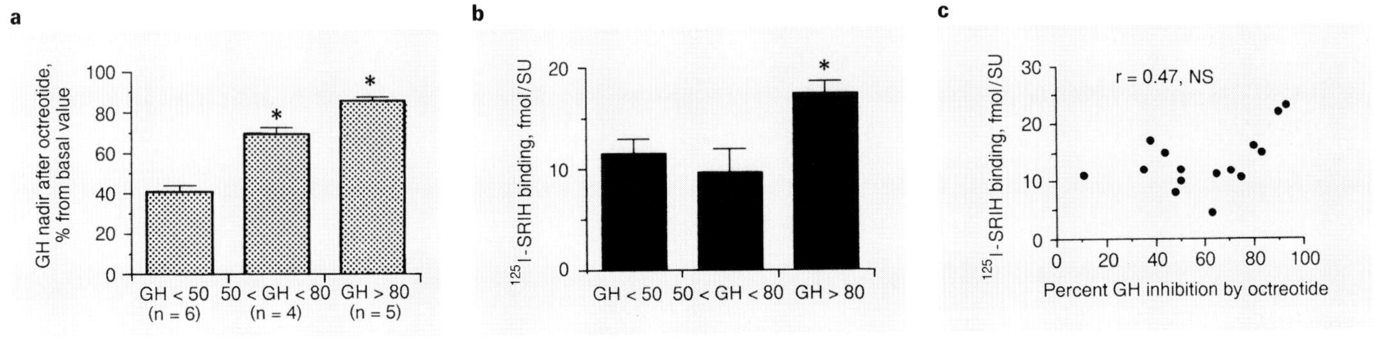

Fig. 2. Correlation between ^{125}I-SRIH binding on the pituitary tumor and in vivo GH response to octreotide in 15 acromegalic patients: (**a**) GH response to octreotide (expressed as % from basal value) and (**b**) ^{125}I-SRIH binding (fmol/surface unit) are compared among the three groups of patients classified according to their response to octreotide (nadir <50% of inhibition, between 50 and 80% and >80% after a single subcutaneous injection of 100 µg octreotide). (**c**) Correlation between ^{125}I-SRIH binding and in vivo GH response to octreotide is shown: * $p < 0.05$.

vidual tumors. The ^{125}I-SRIH-binding site density was reported to be negatively correlated with GH plasma levels before surgery [9]. In these GH-secreting tumors, saturation experiments have revealed a single population of specific binding sites with nanomolar affinity (0.2–1 n*M*). Autoradiographic studies demonstrated that SRIH-binding sites were measurable in 42 out of 43 (98%) of GH-secreting adenomas [34]. These sites are usually homogeneously distributed [33, 35], but a heterogeneous distribution has also been observed in very rare cases [34, 35, and present study].

We measured ^{125}I-SRIH binding in 15 GH-secreting adenomas by quantitative autoradiography using ^{125}I-Tyr$_0$-*D*Trp$_8$-SRIH-14 (780 Ci/m*M*) as previously reported [33]. ^{125}I-SRIH-binding sites were detected on all tumors. Specific binding ranged from 3.8 to 22.2 fmol/surface unit (SU) and the 50% inhibition constant (IC_{50}), calculated from competition with increasing doses of native SRIH, was 7.9 ± 1.6 n*M*. The comparison of ^{125}I-SRIH-specific binding and GH response to octreotide (fig. 2) revealed that mean ^{125}I-SRIH binding was significantly higher in the most sensitive patients, i.e. patients in whom a fall of 80% or more from basal level was observed (^{125}I-SRIH binding: 17.4 ± 1.3 fmol/SU; n = 5), compared to the less responsive patients (GH decrease less than 50% under octreotide: ^{125}I-SRIH binding: 11.6 ± 1.4 fmol/SU; n = 6) and the patients who showed a partial response (GH decrease between 50 and 80% under octreotide, ^{125}I-SRIH binding: 9.6 ± 2.4 fmol/SU; n = 4). However, taken as a whole, the correlation between the

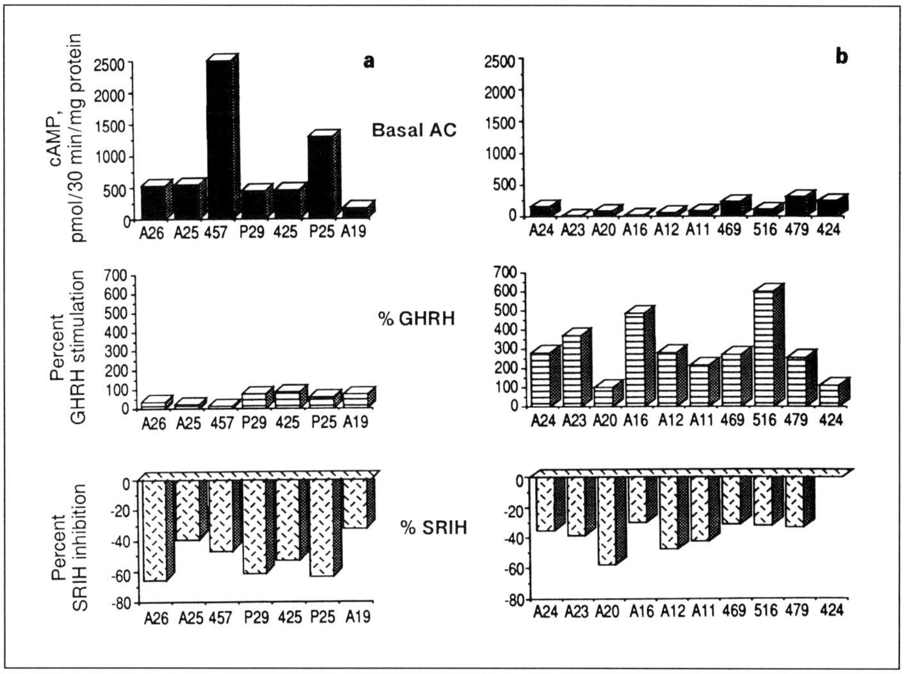

Fig. 3. Basal adenylate cyclase (AC) activity and response to SRIH and GHRH in GH-secreting adenomas. GH-secreting adenomas were classified in two groups according to their basal cyclase activity. In group I (**a**, n = 7) the basal cyclase activity is high (841 ± 306 pmol cAMP/mg protein) and the response to GHRH is low (53 ± 11% stimulation over basal). By contrast, in group II (**b**, n = 10) the basal cyclase activity is lower (252 ± 92 pmol cAMP/mg protein) and the response to GHRH is high (297 ± 48% stimulation over basal). The adenylate cyclase response to SRIH is significantly higher in group I as compared to group II (respective % inhibition of GHRH-stimulated adenylate cyclase activity: 52 ± 5 vs. 34 ± 5, $p < 0.05$).

GH response to octreotide and the ^{125}I-SRIH-binding capacities on the 15 adenomas did not reach statistical significance (r = 0.471).

Adenylate Cyclase Activity Studies

In rat pituitary cell culture, native SRIH-14 and SRIH-28, and various SRIH agonists, including octreotide, inhibit basal and growth hormone releasing hormone (GHRH)-stimulated adenylate cyclase activities [12]. Pretreatment of the cells with pertussis toxin blocks SRIH inhibition of basal and GHRH-stimulated adenylate cyclase as well as SRIH inhibition of GHRH-induced GH secretion. On the other hand, GHRH binding to its cell surface receptor on anterior pituitary results in adenylate cyclase activation [36]. In a subset of GH-secreting tumor, a mutation of α chain of Gs protein that constitutively activates adenylate cyclase has recently been reported [22]. Basal levels of adenylate cyclase are increased in the tumors with mutant Gs protein and no further stimulation of adenylate cyclase activity by GHRH is observed while inhibition of intracellular cyclic AMP levels by SRIH still persists. Furthermore, it was reported that in vivo GH response to SRIH infusion is increased in patients with GH-secreting adenomas with constitutively activated adenylate cyclase [23].

We measured adenylate cyclase activity in 17 GH-secreting adenomas (fig. 3). Seven adenomas displayed significantly higher ($p < 0.05$) basal adenylate cyclase activity as compared to the remaining ten tumors (841 ± 306 vs. 252 ± 92 pmol cAMP/30 min/mg protein). In the seven adenomas with high basal adenylate cyclase activity, stimulation by GHRH was lower (53 ± 11% vs. 297 ± 48%, $p < 0.05$) while SRIH inhibition of intracellular cyclic AMP formation was greater (52 ± 5% vs. 34 ± 5%, $p < 0.05$) than in the ten other adenomas. Although ^{125}I-SRIH-binding sites measured on homogenates of each tumor were higher in the high basal adenylate cyclase adenomas (795 ± 307 vs. 240 ± 94 fmol/mg protein), no direct correlation was apparent between the SRIH inhibition of adenylate cyclase and the amount of binding sites, either on the whole series of adenomas or when they were separated according to their basal adenylate cyclase activities. Thus, the mutation on α_s does not preclude the ability of SRIH agonists to inhibit adenylate cyclase activity.

Correlation between the in vivo Response to SRIH or the SRIH Analog Octreotide, and SRIH Receptors and Adenylate Cyclase Activity in GH-Secreting Adenomas

The first study in acromegalic patients comparing the plasma GH response to synthetic SRIH infusion and the SRIH binding on GH-secreting adenomas was performed on six tumors [19]. In this study, SRIH maximal binding ranged from 41 to 1,018 fmol/mg protein. In all patients but 1 a decrease of at least 47% of GH plasma level was observed during a SRIH infusion of 1 μg/kg/h. The patient who responded minimally (–15%) to SRIH infusion displayed the lowest SRIH maximal binding capacity (41 fmol/mg protein). More recently, Reubi and Landolt [20], using two radioactive ligands developed from SRIH-28 (^{125}I-LTT-SRIH-28) and from octreotide (^{125}I-204-090), concluded to the existence of a correlation between the in vivo response to a single 100-μg subcutaneous injection of octreotide and SRIH receptor autoradiography in 11 acromegalic patients. In this last study, SRIH binding ranged from 30 to 27,120 dpm/mg tissue equivalent with one ligand (^{125}I-204-090) and from 410 to 8,880 dpm/mg tissue equivalent with a second ligand (^{125}I-LTT-SRIH-28). The 2 patients with the lowest ^{125}I-204-090-binding capacities displayed only a partial (although superior to 50% inhibition) response of GH to octreotide. However, this was not observed with ^{125}I-LTT-SRIH-28 for which only 1 patient displayed a low density of binding sites.

From these two studies and our results it sems that differences in SRIH receptor density and affinity on GH-secreting tumors only partially account for the great variability of in vivo responses to SRIH agonists in acromegaly. In very rare cases, GH-secreting adenomas nearly devoid of SRIH-binding sites might indeed be less sensitive to SRIH or octreotide [19, 20]. In our study, a high SRIH receptor density is observed in the most sensitive patients but the less responsive patients (plasma GH decrease after octreotide injection less than 50%) cannot be differentiated from the partially responsive patients (GH decrease from 50 to 80%) on the basis of their ^{125}I-SRIH-binding densities. Alternatively, the partial effect of SRIH agonist therapy is likely to depend on a post-SRIH receptor defect or on intracellular mechanisms not directly dependent upon SRIH actions.

Acknowledgements

We thank Prof. G. Turpin and Prof. A. Warnet (Paris) for providing some of the adenomatous specimens and C. Videau for technical assistance. Photographic work is from INSERM SC6.

References

1 Brazeau P, Vale W, Burgus R, Ling N, Butcher M, River J, Guillemin R: Hypothalamic peptide that inhibits the secretion of immunoreactive pituitary growth hormone. Science 1973; 179:77–79.

2 Hall R, Schally AV, Evered D, Kastin AJ, Mortimer CH, Tunbridge WMG, Besser GM, Coy DH, Goldie DJ, McNeilly AS, Phenekos C, Weightman D: Action of growth-hormone-release inhibitory hormone in healthy men and in acromegaly. Lancet 1973;ii:581–584.

3 Siler TM, Vanderberg G, Yen SSC, Brazeau P, Vale W, Guillemin R: Inhibition of growth hormone release in humans by somatostatin. J Clin Endocrinol Metab 1973;37:632–637.

4 Adams EF, Brajkovich IE, Mashiter K: Hormone secretion by dispersed cell cultures of human pituitary adenomas: Effect of theophylline, thyrotropin-releasing hormone, somatostatin and 2-bromo-α-ergocryptine. J Clin Endocrinol Metab 1979;49:120–126.

5 Kelijman M, Williams TC, Downs TR, Frohman LA: Comparison of the sensitivity of growth hormone secretion to somatostatin in vivo and in vitro in acromegaly. J Clin Endocrinol Metab 1988;67:958–963.

6 Schonbrunn AH, Tashjian AJR: Characterization of functional receptors for somatostatin in rat pituitary cells in culture. J Biol Chem 1978; 253:6473–6483.

7 Reubi JC, Landolt AM: High density of somatostatin receptors in pituitary tumors from acromegalic patients. J Clin Endocrinol Metab 1984;59:1148–1151.

8 Ikuyama S, Nawata H, Kato K, Karashima T, Ibayashi H, Nakagaki H: Specific somatostatin receptors on human pituitary adenoma cell membranes. J Clin Endocrinol Metab 1985;61: 666–671.

9 Moyse E, Le Dafniet M, Epelbaum J, Pagesy P, Peillon F, Kordon C, Enjalbert A: Somatostatin receptors in human growth hormone and prolactin-secreting pituitary adenomas. J Clin Endocrinol Metab 1985;61:98–103.

10 Heisler S, Reisine T, Hook VYH, Axelrod J: Somatostatin inhibits multireceptor stimulation of cyclic AMP formation and corticotropin secretion in mouse pituitary tumor cells. Proc Natl Acad Sci USA 1982;79:6502–6506.

11 Dorflinger L, Schonbrunn A: Somatostatin inhibits vasoactive intestinal peptide-stimulated cyclic adenosine monophosphate accumulation in GH pituitary cells. Endocrinology 1983; 113:1541–1546.

12 Epelbaum J, Enjalbert A, Krantic S, Musset F, Bertrand P, Rasolonjanahary R, Shu C, Kordon C: Somatostatin receptors on pituitary somatotrophs, thyreotrophs and lactotrophs: Pharmacological evidence for loose coupling to adenylate cyclase. Endocrinology 1987;121: 2177–2185.

13 Chen C, Israel JM, Vincent JD: Electrophysiological responses to somatostatin of rat hypophysial cells somatotroph-enriched primary cultures. J Physiol (Lond) 1989;408:493–510.

14 Mollard P, Vacher P, Dufy B, Barker JL: Somatostatin blocks Ca^{2+}-action potential activity in prolactin-secreting pituitary tumor cells through coordinate action of K^+ and Ca^{2+} conductances. Endocrinology 1988;123:721–732.

15 Hanew K, Kokubun M, Sasaki A, Mouri T, Yoshinaga K: The spectrum of pituitary growth hormone responses to pharmacological stimuli in acromegaly. J Clin Endocrinol Metab 1980; 51:292–296.

16 Barkan AL: Acromegaly: Diagnosis and therapy; in Barkan AL (ed): Medical Treatment of Endocrine Tumors. Endocrinology and Metabolism Clinics of North America. Philadelphia, Saunders, 1989, vol 18, pp 277–310.

17 Sassolas G, Harris AG, James-Dedier A: Long-term effect of incremental doses of the somatostatin analog SMS 201-995 in 58 acromegalic patients. J Clin Endocrinol Metab 1990;71: 391–397.

18 Timsit J, Chanson P, Larger E, Duet M, Mosse A, Guillausseau PJ, Harris AG, Moulonguet M, Warnet A, Lubetzki J: The effect of subcutaneous infusion versus subcutaneous injections of a somatostatin analogue (SMS 201-995) on the diurnal GH profile in acromegaly. Acta Endocrinol (Copenh) 1987;116:108–112.

19 Ikuyama S, Nawata H, Kato KI, Ibayashi H, Nakagaki H: Plasma growth hormone responses to somatostatin (SRIH) and SRIH receptors in pituitary adenomas in acromegalic patients. J Clin Endocrinol Metab 1986;62: 729–733.
20 Reubi JC, Landolt AM: The growth hormone response to octreotide in acromegaly correlate with adenoma somatostatin receptor status. J Clin Endocrinol Metab 1989;68:844–850.
21 Vallar L, Spada A, Giannattasio G: Altered Gs and adenylate cyclase activity in human GH-secreting pituitary adenomas. Nature 1987; 330:566–568.
22 Lyons J, Landis CA, Harsh G, Vallar L, Grünewald K, Feichtinger H, Duh QY, Clark OH, Kawasaki E, Bourne HR, McCormick F: Two G protein oncogenes in human endocrine tumors. Science 1990;249:655–659.
23 Spada A, Arosio M, Bochicchio D, Bazzoni N, Vallar L, Bassetti M, Faglia G: Clinical, biochemical, and morphological correlates in patients bearing growth hormone-secreting pituitary tumors with or without constitutively active adenyl cyclase. J Clin Endocrinol Metab 1990;71:1421–1426.
24 Lamberts SWJ, Uitterlinden P, Schuijff PC, Klijn JGM: Therapy of acromegaly with Sandostatin: The predictive value of an acute test, the value of serum SmC measurements in dose adjustment and the definition of a biochemical cure. Clin Endocrinol 1988;29:411–420.
25 James RA, White MC, Moller N, Chatterjee S, Hall K, Kendall-Taylor P: Continuous infusion of octreotide in acromegaly. Lancet 1989;ii: 1083–1087.
26 Harris AG, Prestele H, Herold K: Long-term efficacy of Sandostatin (SMS 201-995, octreotide) in 178 acromegalic patients. Results from the International Multicentre Acromegaly Study Group; in Lamberts SWJ (ed): Sandostatin in the Treatment of Acromegaly. New York, Springer, 1988, pp 117–125.
27 Srikant CB, Patel YC: Characterization of pituitary membrane receptors for somatostatin in the rat. Endocrinology 1982;110:2138–2146.
28 Aguilera G, Parker DS: Pituitary somatostatin receptors: Characterization by binding with a nondegradable peptide analogue. J Biol Chem 1982;257:1134–1137.
29 Enjalbert A, Tapia-Arancibia L, Rieurort M, Moyse E, Kordon C, Epelbaum J: Somatostatin receptors on rat anterior pituitary membranes. Endocrinology 1982;110:1634–1640.
30 Reubi JC, Perrin M, Rivier J, Vale W: High affinity binding sites for somatostatin to rat pituitary. Biochem Biophy Res Commun 1982; 105:1538–1545.
31 Enjalbert A, Rasolonjanahary R, Moyse E, Kordon C, Epelbaum J: Guanine nucleotide sensitivity of ^{125}I-iodo-NTyr somatostatin binding in rat adenohypophysis and cerebral cortex. Endocrinology 1983;113:822–824.
32 Polak M, Bertherat J, Li JY, Kujas M, le Dafniet M, Weizani H, Van Effenterre R, Epelbaum J, Turpin G: A human TSH-secreting adenoma: Endocrine, biochemical and morphological studies. Evidence of somatostatin receptors by using quantitative autoradiography. Clinical and biological improvement by SMS 201-995 treatment. Acta Endocrinol (Copenh) 1991;124:479–486.
33 Bertherat J, Brue T, Enjalbert A, Gunz G, Rasolonjanahary R, Warnet A, Jacquet P, Epelbaum J: Somatostatin receptors on thyrotropin-secreting pituitary adenomas: Comparison with the inhibitory effects of octreotide upon in vivo and in vitro hormonal secretions. J Clin Endocrinol Metab 1992;75:540–547.
34 Lamberts SW, Krenning EP, Reubi JC: The role of somatostatin and its analogs in the diagnosis and treatment of tumors. Endocr Rev 1991;12:450–482.
35 Reubi JC, Heitz PU, Landolt AM: Visualization of somatostatin receptors and correlation with immunoreactive growth hormone and prolactin in human pituitary adenomas: Evidence for different tumor subclasses. J Clin Endocrinol Metab 1987;65:65–73.
36 Bilezijkian LM, Vale WW: Stimulation of adenosine 3′,5′-monophosphate production by growth hormone-releasing factor and its inhibition by somatostatin in anterior pituitary cells in vitro. Endocrinology 1983;113:1726–1731.

Note Added in Proof

Since submission of this paper, the cloning and sequencing of genes encoding three SRIH receptors of 369-, 391- [Yamada Y, Post SR, Wang K, Tager HW, Bell GI, Seino: Proc Natl Acad Sci USA 89:251–255, and Kluxen FW, Bruns C, Lübbert H: Proc Natl Acad Sci USA 89:4618–4622] and 428- [Yasuda K, Rens-Damiano S, Breder CD, Law SF, Saper CB, Reisine T, Bell GI: J Biol Chem 267:20422–20428, and Meyerhoff W, Wulfsen I, Schönrock C, Fehr S, Richter D: Proc Natl Acad Sci USA 89:10267–10271] amino acids have been reported. The three receptors are members of the seven transmembrane domains superfamily of G-protein coupled receptors. The two smaller ones display equivalent affinities for the two endogenous peptides of the somatostatin family (i.e. SRIH-14 and SRIH-28) while the longer one is slightly SRIH-28-preferring. It remains to be demonstrated which of these receptors (or some others awaiting to be cloned) is preferentially expressed in GH-secreting pituitary adenomas. These recent findings add an interesting level of diversity in the mechanisms of resistance to SRIH analog therapy.

Horm Res 1992;38:100–104

D. Joubert
B. Mouhieddine
C. Benlot
L. Levy
F. Peillon

INSERM U223, Paris, France

Autocrine and Paracrine Effects of Peptides on Human Pituitary Cells

Key Words
Somatostatin
Growth hormone
Pituitary adenomas

Abstract
In contrast to normal human pituitaries, GH-secreting adenomas cannot process in vivo ProSRIH whereas they do it in vitro. The existence of an endogenous factor able to inhibit ProSRIH processing in vivo was postulated and such a role was analyzed for GHRH. Results showed that when GH adenomas are incubated in vitro with GHRH $10^{-8}M$, their ProSRIH contents are decreased, percent inhibition being negatively correlated to the amount of endogenously released GHRH. When incubation is performed in the presence of GHRH antibody in order to block the effect of endogenous GHRH, ProSRIH content is increased. The same effects are observed on SRIH release: inhibition by GHRH, stimulation by GHRH antibody. Normal rabbit serum had no effect. It may therefore be concluded that the absence of ProSRIH maturation observed in adenomas in vivo may be the consequence of the GHRH release that is known to be higher from GH adenomas than from normal pituitaries.

Introduction

Paracrine and autocrine regulations are now recognized to be potentially involved in the control of pituitary hormonal release [1, 2]. They implicate several peptides including vasoactive intestinal peptide (VIP) [3], thyroliberin (TRH) [4, 5], Growth hormone (GH)-releasing hormone (GHRH) [6], somatostatin (SRIH) [7], substance P [8] or neuropeptide Y [8]. Studies performed on rat and on human tissues have demonstrated the capacity of the pituitary to synthesize these peptides [9–11] as well as to release them in vitro [8]. Immunocytochemistry brought some information on the localization of these substances, which may either be colocalized with a pituitary hormone [12, 13] or be in specific cells as it is for SRIH [14]. Messenger RNAs as well as translation products are not different from what has already been characterized in the hypothalamus, and arises now as a new concept, called by Krisch [15] 'the paraneuron concept' which compares in many points neurons and some endocrine cells with a common embryologic origin, the neural crest. Both neurons and paraneurons produce the same substances, store them in vesicles and release them upon specific stimulation.

In this paper, we will focus our attention on the regulations involving SRIH and GHRH synthesized in the

D. Joubert, MD
Centre CNRS-INSERM de Pharmacologie et d'Endocrinologie
rue de la Cardonille
F–34094 Montpellier Cedex 5 (France)

0301–0163/92/0382–0100
$2.75/0

human pituitary itself and in particular on the involvement of GHRH in the alteration in ProSRIH processing observed in GH-secreting adenomas [16].

Materials and Methods

Patients

GH-secreting adenomas, obtained from acromegalic patients with high plasma GH (range 10–150 µg/l, > 5 µg/l normal subjects) were collected in the operating room after transsphenoidal adenomectomy. Normal pituitaries were obtained 4–8 h after death from subjects (range 20–80 years old) with no evidence of neuroendocrine disorders.

Fragments of adenomas and pituitaries were used immediately in perifusion studies, others were frozen for quantification of SRIH, GHRH or ProSRIH tissue contents. The rest was used for light microscopy and immunocytochemistry. Diagnosis before surgery was established on clinical, biological and radiological criteria. Morphological and immunocytochemical studies confirmed the diagnosis.

Perifusion Studies

Basal GH, SRIH and GHRH release profiles were observed using this procedure: fragments (15 mg) of pituitary tissues collected post-mortem or mechanically dispersed cells (1 × 10^6 cells) from GH-secreting adenomas were perifused in an isolated chamber at 37 °C containing 0.4 g Bio-Gel P2. The perifusion medium contained 118 mmol/l NaCl, 4.7 mmol/l KCl, 1.18 mmol/l KH_2PO_4, 2.5 mmol/l $CaCl_2$, 25 mmol/l $NaHCO_3$, 1.18 mmol/l $MgSO_4$ and 14 mmol/l glucose supplemented with 5 g/l BSA and a mixture of amino acids. The medium was constantly gassed with CO_2-O_2 (5-95%). Fractions (1 ml) were collected every 2 min and immediately frozen at –20 °C until GH, SRIH and GHRH assays.

Static Incubation

Regulation of SRIH release and of ProSRIH synthesis by GHRH was observed in static incubation: fragments (300 mg) were incubated for 4 h in the absence or presence of GHRH (10^{-8} *M*), GHRH antibody (final dilution 1/1,000; generous gift of M.C. Thonon, Rouen) or rabbit preimmune serum (final dilution 1/1,000). At the end of incubation, fragments were recovered after centrifugation and extracted with 2 *M* acetic acid for further analysis of their GHRH, SRIH and ProSRIH contents. Medium was frozen until GHRH and SRIH assays.

Tissue Extraction (SRIH and GHRH) and Sephadex G-50 Filtration (ProSRIH)

Normal and tumoral pituitaries were boiled for 5 min in 2 *M* acetic acid, homogenized (1:10, w/v) and then kept frozen overnight. After thawing, homogenates were centrifuged at 2,000 *g* for 20 min. Proteins were assayed in pellets by the methods of Lowry. Aliquots of supernatants were lyophilized for their GHRH and SRIH contents. The rest was loaded on a Sephadex G-50 column (90 × 2 cm) and eluted at 4 °C with 5.2 *M* acetic acid for their ProSRIH contents. Fractions (1.7 ml) were collected at 10-min intervals, lyophilized and assayed for SRIH by radioimmunoassay (RIA). Immunoreactive fractions were further analyzed by HPLC and Western blot in order to characterize ProSRIH [16].

Table 1. SRIH and GHRH contents of normal human pituitaries (n = 6) and of GH adenomas (n = 11) in pg/mg proteins

	Normal pituitaries	GH adenomas
SRIH	11.3 ± 4.6	not detectable
GHRH	564 ± 135	220 ± 26

Hormone Assays

IR-SRIH, IR-GHRH and GH were assayed as previously described [4]. The SRIH antibody recognizes ProSRIH as the SRIH 1-14 sequence is in the C-terminal part of the molecule. ProSRIH is expressed as equivalent SRIH 1-14.

Results and Discussion

GH-Secreting Adenomas Cannot Process in vivo ProSRIH

GHRH and SRIH tissue content quantification indicated that whereas both normal pituitaries and GH adenomas contain GHRH, SRIH is not detectable in GH adenomas (table 1).

Normal pituitaries (rat and human) contain SRIH in equivalent amounts, comparable to what has been published by Morel and co-workers. However, the absence of SRIH in adenomas is not concomitant to the absence of mRNAs encoding preproSRIH. Indeed, two different studies from two different laboratories have shown the presence of these mRNAs in all GH adenomas. Quantification of ProSRIH tissue contents indicated that mRNAs encoding preproSRIH are translated in only 50% of adenomas and that ProSRIH adenoma contents are highly variable in the remaining 50%. In addition, the absence of ProSRIH maturation in vivo in GH adenomas is further evidenced by the absence of detectable SRIH release at the beginning of the perifusion.

GH-Secreting Adenomas Process in vitro ProSRIH

The absence of ProSRIH processing in vivo is not an irreversible phenomenon. Indeed, these tumoral cells are able to release SRIH in vitro after a variable lag time and are able to synthesize ProSRIH in vitro.

Figure 1 depicts the profile of SRIH release from a GH adenoma. SRIH is released in this experiment after 1 h of perifusion (this lag time may be as long as 4 h) and is

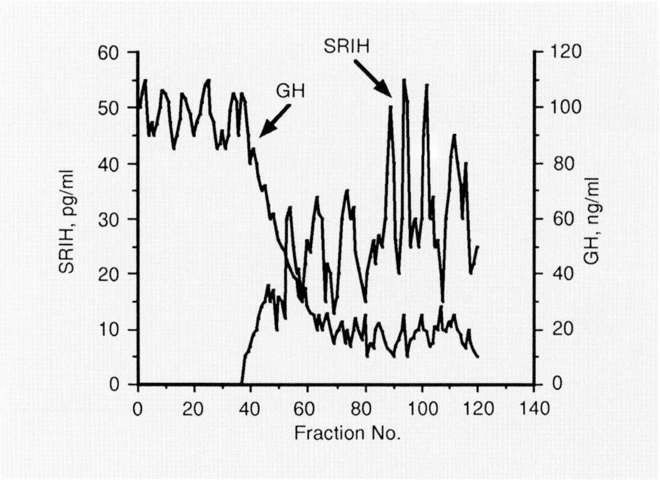

Fig. 1. GH and SRIH releases from a perifused GH adenoma. Fractions (1 ml) were collected every 2 min and frozen until assayed for their GH and SRIH contents.

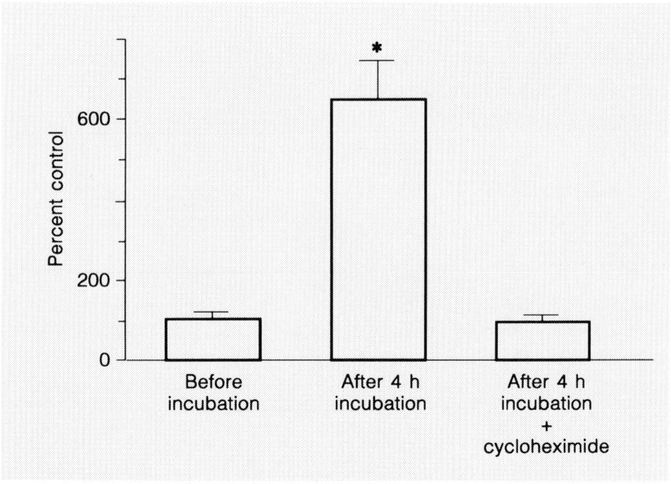

Fig. 2. In vitro synthesis of ProSRIH in GH adenomas (n = 3) incubated for 4 h with or without cycloheximide (10^{-5} *M*). * = $p < 0.01$.

Table 2. GHRH release from normal pituitaries (n = 4) and from GH adenomas (n = 5) in pg/mg proteins (range)

Normal pituitaries	GH adenomas
40–372	1,980–6,760

always concomitant to a significant decrease of GH release.

When GH-secreting adenomas are incubated for 4 h ProSRIH content is significantly higher than before incubation (fig. 2), the increase in ProSRIH content being abolished when incubation is performed in the presence of cycloheximide (10^{-5} *M*).

The fact that GH adenomas process in vitro ProSRIH indicates that the alteration of ProSRIH processing in vivo does not result from a deficiency in the enzymes involved in ProSRIH maturation. Rather it may suggest the presence, in vivo, of an endogenous factor that inhibits this processing. Several arguments argue in favor of such a role for GHRH.

The first argument is the presence of GHRH in all GH-secreting adenomas (table 1). The second one is that GHRH is released in vitro in higher amounts from adenomas than from normal pituitaries (table 2), and the third one is that SRIH release appears in the perifusion medium only when that of GHRH has disappeared [6]. We indeed demonstrated that GHRH is an endogenous factor able to inhibit ProSRIH maturation and SRIH release at the level of the pituitary itself.

Effect of GHRH on ProSRIH Synthesis

When a GH adenoma is incubated in the presence of GHRH 10^{-8} *M*, its ProSRIH content is decreased when compared to the control incubation (fig. 3). The percentage of inhibition is negatively correlated to the amount of GHRH that is endogenously released by the pituitary tissue itself (estimated by RIA quantification in the medium of the control incubation; fig. 3). This indicates that the more GHRH is released, the lower will be the effect produced by exogenous GHRH. It also suggests that endogenous GHRH is capable of inhibiting pituitary ProSRIH synthesis in vitro. Indeed, when adenoma fragments are incubated in the presence of GHRH antibody (1/1,000 final dilution), ProSRIH content is significantly increased as compared to control incubation.

Effect of GHRH on SRIH Release

Inhibition of ProSRIH synthesis by GHRH parallels an inhibition of SRIH release (fig. 4) and, as it was observed for ProSRIH, incubation with GHRH antibody has an opposite effect. Indeed, GHRH antibody induces a significant increase of SRIH release, which is not repro-

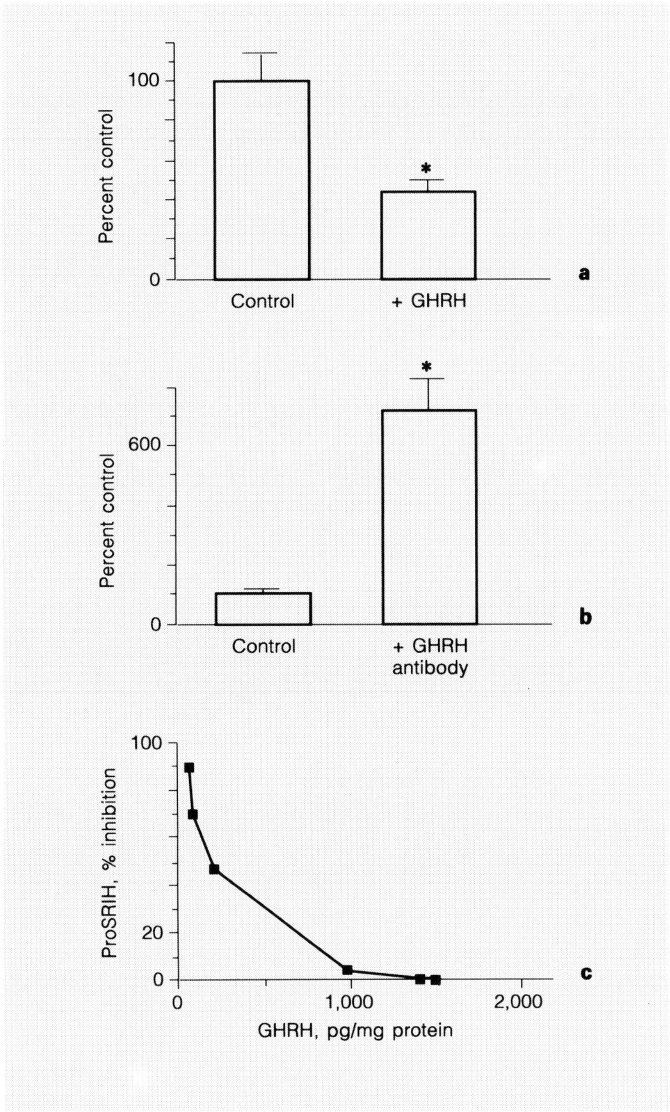

3

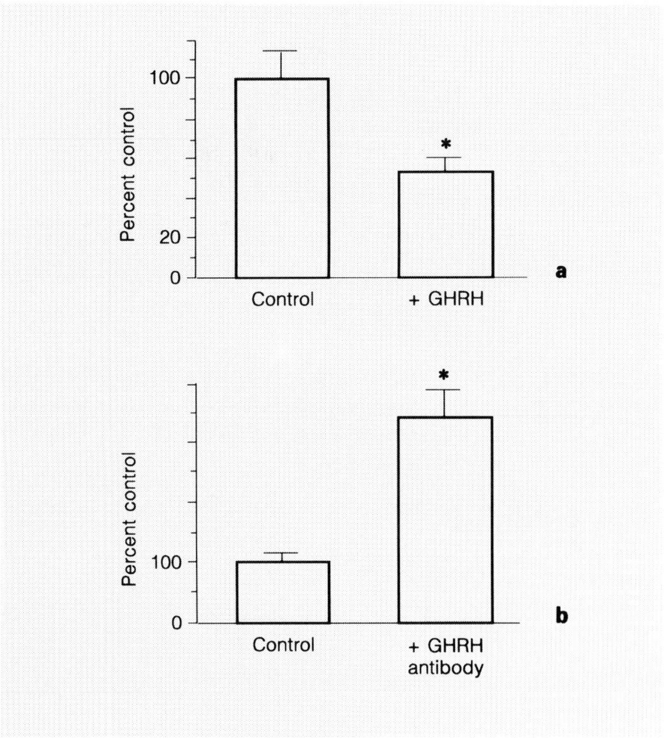

4

Fig. 3. Effect of GHRH (10^{-8} *M*) (**a**) and of the GHRH antibody (1/1,000 final dilution) (**b**) on ProSRIH content of GH adenomas incubated for 4 h. * = $p < 0.01$. Negative relationship between the percent inhibition induced by exogenous GHRH on ProSRIH content and the amount of GHRH endogenously released (**c**).

Fig. 4. Effect of (**a**) GHRH (10^{-8} *M*) and of (**b**) GHRH antibody (1/1,000 final dilution) on SRIH release from GH adenomas (n = 4).

duced by incubation with normal rabbit serum used at 1/1,000 final dilution (fig. 4).

Inhibition of ProSRIH synthesis and SRIH release by GHRH (exogenous and endogenous) is not a specific effect observed only on GH adenomas. It is also observed on normal human pituitaries: significant increase in ProSRIH content and SRIH release in the presence of GHRH antibody and inhibition in the presence of GHRH.

Overall, these results indicate a relationship between GHRH and pituitary SRIH. The negative regulation that GHRH exerts on SRIH is found both in adenomas and in normal pituitaries. However, the fact that adenomas release higher amounts of GHRH than normal tissues may be related to the absence of ProSRIH maturation in these tumoral cells. Indeed the inhibition that GHRH exerts on SRIH in the normal tissue is, in adenomas, amplified and results in the absence of SRIH, which can no longer inhibit GH release and thus leads finally to a potentialization of GH stimulation by GHRH. This alteration in the equilibrium between autocrine or paracrine regulation involving pituitary GHRH and SRIH may participate in GH hypersecretion if not in cell proliferation as well; one has to keep in mind that both peptides are able to regulate somatotroph's proliferation and one accepts now as an evidence that autocrine or paracrine regulations may play a role in tumorigenesis.

References

1 Denef C, Baes M, Schramme C: Paracrine interactions in the anterior pituitary: Role in the regulation of prolactin and growth hormone secretion. Front Endocrinol 1986;9:115–148.

2 Jones TH, Brown BL, Dobson PRM: Paracrine control of anterior pituitary hormone secretion. J Endocrinol 1990;127:5–13.

3 Lam KSL, Lechan RM, Minamitani N, Segerson TP, Reichlin S: Vasoactive intestinal peptide in the anterior pituitary is increased in hypothyrodism. Endocrinology 1989;124:1077–1084.

4 Le Dafniet M, Levebvre P, Barret A, et al: Normal and adenomatous human pituitaries secrete thyrotropin-releasing hormone in vitro: Modulation by dopamine, haloperidol and somatostatin. J Clin Endocrinol Metab 1990;71:480–486.

5 Bruhn TO, Bolduc TG, Maclean DB, Jackson IMD: ProTRH peptides are synthesized and secreted by anterior pituitary cells in long-term culture. Endocrinology 1991;129:556–558.

6 Joubert (Bression) D, Benlot C, Lagoguey A, et al: Normal and growth hormone (GH)-secreting adenomatous human pituitaries release somatostatin and GH-releasing hormone. J Clin Endocrinol Metab 1989;68:572–577.

7 Benlot C, Pagesy P, Peillon F, Joubert-Bression D: Growth hormone-releasing hormone and somatostatin in normal and tumoral human pituitaries. Peptides 1991;12:945–950.

8 O'Halloran D, Jones PM, Ghatei MA, Domin J, Bloom SR: The regulation of neuropeptide expression in rat anterior pituitary following chronic manipulation of estrogen status: A comparison between substance P, neuropeptide Y, neurotensin and vasoactive intestinal peptide. Endocrinology 1990;127:1463–1469.

9 Arnaout MA, Garthwaite TL, Martinson DR, Hagen TC: Vasoactive intestinal polypeptide is synthesized in anterior pituitary tissue. Endocrinology 1986;119:2052–2057.

10 Pagesy P, Li JY, Rentier-Delrue F, et al: Evidence of preprosomatostatin (preproSRIH) messenger ribonucleic acid (mRNA) in human normal and tumoral anterior pituitary gland. Mol Endocrinol 1989;3:1289–1294.

11 Nagy G, Mulchahey JJ, Neill JD: Autocrine control of prolactin secretion by vasoactive intestinal peptide. Endocrinology 1988;122:364–366.

12 Köves K, Gottschall PE, Görcs T, Scammel JG, Arimura A: Presence of immunoreactive vasoactive intestinal polypeptide in anterior pituitary of normal male and long-term estrogen-treated female rats: A light microscopic immunohistochemical study. Endocrinology 1990;126:1756–1763.

13 Hsu D, Riskind PN, Hedley-Whyte ET: Vasoactive intestinal peptide in the human pituitary gland and adenomas. Am J Pathol 1989;135:329–338.

14 Li JY, Pagesy P, Berthet M, et al: Somatostatin cells in human somatotropic adenomas. Virchows Arch [A] 1992;420:95–101.

15 Krisch B: The hypothalamo-hypophyseal complex: A paradigm of the paraneuron concept. Arch Histol Cytol 1989;52:365–373.

16 Levy L, Bourdais J, Mouhieddine B, et al: Presence and characterization of the somatostatin precursor in normal human pituitaries and in GH-secreting adenomas. J Clin Endocrinol Metab, in press.